Managing Your Migraine

Managing Your Migraine

A Migraine Sufferer's Practical Guide

by

Susan L. Burks, MEd

Foreword by

Fred D. Sheftell, MD

 Humana Press, Totowa, New Jersey

Dedication

This work is dedicated to all those who suffer from migraine and are misunderstood.

The information and recommendations in *Managing Your Migraine* are firmly grounded in the medical literature, and/or the author's and her sources clinical experience, and so are relevant and appropriate in most cases. For specific information concerning your personal medical condition, it is suggested that you consult a physician. The names of organizations appearing in this book are given for informational purposes only.

© 1994 Humana Press Inc.
999 Riverview Drive, Suite 208
Totowa, New Jersey 07512

Printed in the United States of America. 10 9 8 7 6 5 4 3

Library of Congress Cataloging-in-Publication Data

Burks, Susan L.
    Managing your migraine; a migraine sufferer's practical guide/
            by Susan L. Burks; foreword by Fred D. Sheftell.
                    p. cm.
            Includes index.
            ISBN 0-89603-277-9 (hardcover) ISBN 0-89603-324-4 (paperback)
            1. Migraine—Popular works. I. Title.
            RC392.B78   1994   94-4712
            616.8'57–dc20   CIP

Foreword

Migraine sufferers and those of us involved in treating them are indebted to Susan Burks for her invaluable contribution, *Managing Your Migraine*. One of the many unique features of this book is that it is authored by a migraine sufferer, providing the reader with a perspective that is unlikely to be gained from books on the same subject written by physicians. As close as I am to migraine patients in my daily work, I do not suffer from the disorder myself, and thus my perspective is from the "outside in." Ms. Burks, on the other hand, chronicles her own battles with migraine and shares the many personal discoveries she has made—borne out of her pain, her unceasing efforts to conquer it, and her desire to help her daughter.

Ms. Burks' personal trials and tribulations, as well as her successes and failures, clearly show that one cannot take a "cookbook" approach to managing migraine. Rather, highly individualized combinations of medical and nonmedical interventions are called for.

The more education that is available about migraine, the better we can dispel the many myths and half truths surrounding it. In spite of the fact that, in the United States alone, 18% of women and 6% of men suffer from migraine, the vast majority have never been diagnosed as having the disorder and have never received appropriate treatment. For physicians, there is little formal education on migraine and related disorders, both during medical school and in postgraduate training. My fellow medical students and I certainly learned about the ominous causes of headache, such as brain tumors, aneurysms, infections, and so forth, but unfortunately we did *not* receive the training necessary to diagnose and treat the most common headache disorders. Those of us who have developed an interest in migraine have had to learn largely through our own efforts and independent study. In following the same path, Ms. Burks has developed considerable expertise in the subject, which she shares with us in this book. Her book is living proof that one does not need to be a medical professional to understand a complex medical disorder and to use that knowledge to help oneself and others.

Our working relationship in completing the book has been especially enjoyable for me. In fact, I think our collaboration embodies the concept of "partnership" between physician and patient outlined in the book's first chapter. I am a firm believer that mutuality of effort on the part of patient and physician is absolutely essential in achieving successful management and restoration of quality of life. Those sufferers who are willing to take responsibility and help themselves have a far better outcome than those who rely completely on their physicians for help. I see this reality as the most important "take-home" message of our book. Thus, *Managing Your Migraine* should serve as a guide for self-learning and should be shared with your physician as a working template in seeking relief.

In summary, *Managing Your Migraine* is a comprehensive treatment of the subject—one that offers a wide variety of practical tips in regard to medications, diet, lifestyle, and guides to self-help. Ms. Burks' research has been extensive. The dietary information she provides is particularly comprehensive, including not only which foods should be eliminated, but also suggesting various levels of dietary restriction and explaining which foods are appropriate for whom.

This book should be required reading for patients, their families, and their physicians alike.

Fred D. Sheftell, MD, Codirector
The New England Center for Headache
Stamford, CT

Preface

If you have done much reading about migraines, you may have noticed that most of the books and articles are written either by physicians or by objective medical reporters. In my wide reading on the topic, I recall only three books and two articles actually written by fellow migraine sufferers; none of these were both comprehensive and up-to-date. Of course I recognize the value of getting the medical practitioners' perspective and expertise, but I also believe there is room for another perspective—that of an actual headache sufferer.

Thus, *Managing Your Migraine* is written primarily to share the results of my own long struggle against migraine—not to weep and wail and gain sympathy, although I do admit to feeling a certain satisfaction that there are many others who understand the migraine ordeal. In sharing my successes and failures in understanding and treating the disorder, combined with the knowledge I have gained from extensive research, I hope to provide you, my companion sufferer, a measure of support—and with any luck to spare you some pain.

So that you will better understand the context of *Managing Your Migraine*, please allow me to include here a note about my own experience of the illness. I am a 53-year-old woman whose migraine attacks struck with a vengeance during my 35th year. Looking back with the benefit of current knowledge, I realize that I had in fact experienced very mild and infrequent attacks as a child and young teen, but for well over a decade I had been totally symptom free. Not only did I not have *severe* headaches, I had no headaches at all!

From ages 35 to 49, however, my condition gradually worsened until finally I was experiencing pain, or at least discomfort, most of the time, and was feeling as if I had lost control of my life. My actual attacks involved several days of dizziness, lightheadedness, head and often back pain, nausea and vomiting, alternating chills and sweats, and sleeplessness. Then, when the acute attack subsided, hangover symptoms followed, sometimes lasting until the beginning of the next attack. Because I was so sensitive to chemical fumes, dust, common foods, and preservatives, many everyday situations literally became hazardous to both my physical and emotional health.

Certainly every area of my life suffered: I became a grumpy, disagreeable wife and mother and began to shy away from involvement in new activities and relationships, either because I did not feel up to them physically or emotionally or because I feared making commitments that I might be unable to keep. In short, I became one miserable person before I finally began to realize that I needed to make an all-out effort to help myself. I am still not cured, but I have come a very long way. My last disabling attack occurred more than three years ago, and the occasional headaches I do continue to experience are relatively mild.

The story of how I got from there to here unfolds gradually in *Managing Your Migraine* along with the fruits of my research, greatly aided by my medical editor, Dr. Fred Sheftell, Cofounder and Codirector of the New England Center for Headache in Stamford, Connecticut.

One of the strongest motivating factors compelling me to conduct in-depth research and finally to put it all together in the form of a book was the fact that my daughter also suffers from migraines. My parental instinct inspired me to try to protect her from as much pain as is humanly possible.

My perspective is, I will admit, different, not only because it stems from personal struggle and maternal concern, but also because it reflects my biases. And I do want to share with you, up-front, the nature and extent of those biases that I consider significant.

I assume migraine to stem from a genetic, biological predisposition, meaning that the tendency toward the disorder is both inherited and physical in nature; this tendency probably reflects a central nervous system defect. At the same time I also assume—because of my personal experience, contact with other sufferers, and my in-depth research—that certain environmental influences can either lessen or worsen such a tendency, sometimes quite dramatically. For me that's the really good news: Often a migraineur can raise his or her threshold for experiencing painful attacks, resulting in either less frequent or less severe symptoms, or both; some sufferers even succeed in eliminating attacks completely.

I am writing *Managing Your Migraine* in the admirable tradition of the late Norman Cousins, whose spirit in relating to chronic illness I greatly admire. Like Cousins, I firmly believe in a person's ability and right to direct his or her own treatment, in partnership with an empathetic physician and other appropriate health-care professionals. Therefore I affirm the wise notion that a layperson must first become a knowledgeable medical consumer to be in a position to assume that responsibility.

I began my research in an attempt to relieve my personal misery; soon I realized that a significant and potentially dangerous gap exists between the latest research findings and what the typical doctor offers the average patient. In his radio talk-show, medical journalist Dr. Dean Edell often expresses concern about this lag time, noting that the practicing physician devotes very little, if any, time to reading medical journals or otherwise keeping abreast of the latest research findings. This situation strikes me as one in which no one is minding the store; the patient inaccurately assumes that his or her physician is providing the most up-to-date treatment, but apparently there is no strong incentive or convenient opportunity for many physicians to do so. I am suggesting that if you, as a migraineur, fail to keep up with the latest research yourself, then there is no assurance that anyone else will do it for you. In *Managing Your Migraine* I suggest some avenues for becoming a better-informed medical consumer.

Also like my role model Cousins, I prefer the greatest possible reliance on nondrug interventions in treating any illness, with serious emphasis on lifestyle change and minimal, if any, use of either prescription or over-the-counter medications. But please don't take that statement to mean that I am against using drugs. Not at all—I simply believe in keeping them as a last resort. In migraine treatment these nondrug strategies include maintaining regular sleeping and eating schedules, modifying dietary intake, changing the way stress is perceived and handled, implementing a regimen of regular aerobic exercise, and avoiding certain aggravating chemicals and medications.

A warning: If you do not, for any reason, wish to assume primary responsibility for the management of your illness, then this book is not for you. If you lean toward leaving treatment decisions solely in the hands of your physician or are searching for a magic pill to cure your migraines, then you probably will not benefit from my research and experiences. The migraine management program presented here requires from you a moderate amount of motivation, thoughtful consideration, flexibility, time, and energy.

My own educational background, in combination with an unusual amount of available time and motivation, have allowed me to pursue a greater understanding of migraine than the average layperson is in a position to do. In completing my master's degree in counseling at the College of William and Mary, I learned both how to evaluate research data and how to help others change their behavior. The result of my labors is a practical, down-to-earth book. (And because I fully recognize the seriousness of the subject of migraine, I feel free at times to take a somewhat flippant approach to it.)

Managing Your Migraine is meant as a complement to professional hands-on medical care, rather than as a substitute for it. I am not a medical professional, and neither the publisher nor I assumes responsibility for the unforeseen consequences of any specific individual application of the information presented herein. I am consistently careful to differentiate between research findings, opinions of experts, and my own personal experiences and opinions; I leave it to you to note and respond appropriately to such distinctions. As Chapter 1 emphasizes, I recommend that you do not even continue reading beyond the end of that chapter unless and until you have

(1) been diagnosed as suffering from migraines; and (2) formed a working relationship with a competent, caring physician.

I wish you success in traversing your personal migraine tightrope. My own journey has been a most frustrating one. Finally, I have reestablished my equilibrium. My hope is that *Managing Your Migraine* will help you maintain or regain your balance on the narrow, swaying surface of the migraineur's tightrope, during what is almost certain to be a challenging journey.

Susan L. Burks

Acknowledgments

I express my warmest gratitude to:

My "family editorial committee," my aunt Pauline Drawver and my daughter Stephanie Burks, both of whom conscientiously corrected my errors of punctuation, grammar, and spelling, and to Stephanie, who provided invaluable technical assistance with the word-processing tasks as well.

The volunteer readers (all migraineurs of varying degrees themselves) Shirley Stein, Joe Barrett, Freda Bolding, Elena Barr, Julie Walls, and Mercedes Kassel, who improved the organization, readability, and usefulness of these pages immensely.

Dr. Sheftell, my medical consultant, who has been extremely encouraging and helpful. Indeed, if more physicians shared his attitude and expertise, living with migraine would be a great deal easier, and I might never have felt the need to write this book at all!

The librarians who patiently assisted with my research, especially Betsy Bishop, the medical librarian at Mary Immaculate Hospital, Newport News, and Peggy Cook, interlibrary loan coordinator at my local branch of the Newport News Public Library.

The typists and proofreaders who helped me save my wrists and my eyes for another day.

And, last but by no means least, my husband Harold, who bought me a wonderful new printer, took up the slack at home, and lovingly held my hand.

Now I understand the reason authors traditionally become so emotive at this point. I really do not believe I would or could have written this book without your help and support.

Thank You All!

Contents

Chapter 1

Where To Turn/What To Ask For

A Good Diagnosis: *Necessary But Not Sufficient*

If you are experiencing headaches painful enough to interfere significantly with your lifestyle and have not yet obtained a diagnosis, then you need to consult a physician right away. For a person suffering severe headaches, an accurate diagnosis is medically essential. The possibility that your headaches might be caused by a life-threatening condition, such as a brain tumor or a stroke, although extremely small, should never be dismissed out of hand. Sometimes headaches are only symptoms of underlying medical conditions—such as high blood pressure, thyroid imbalance, or eye disease—all of which can certainly benefit from proper treatment.

If the headache constitutes a primary disorder, rather than signaling the presence of some other disease, an accurate diagnosis is critical to successful treatment. The bottom line is clear: Neither you nor your physician will know how to manage your headaches until you know what type they are.

If you already have a trusted family doctor, then starting with him or her makes sense. If you have not formed such a relationship, then you may want to invest some serious time and effort in locating a competent primary-care physician. Relying on emergency-room physicians or walk-in clinics for either diagnosis or ongoing care is not a good idea. Two national organizations, the National Headache Foundation and the American Council for Headache Education, will provide you with a list of physicians in your area who are interested in headache treatment. For contact information on these organizations, see the section on "Other Resources" near the end of this chapter.

Here are some ideas for maximizing the chances of an accurate diagnosis: Go to a headache clinic if one with a good reputation is convenient, or choose a doctor who has a special interest in treating headaches. This might be a family practitioner, an internist, or a neurologist. Ask around, but do not assume that all neurologists automatically possess such an interest. Although these specialists are supposedly qualified to diagnose and treat headaches, some seem satisfied with ruling out the existence of brain tumors and

1

then perhaps offering a prescription—not even an approximation of the holistic treatment many sufferers desire.

The Headache Workup: *What to Expect*

Your doctor's first priority will probably be to give you a thorough physical examination if you have not had one recently. This likely will include checking significant neurological functions, such as balance, coordination, and reflexes—including how your eyes track—as well as ordering some blood work. Depending on the outcome of your office exam and blood work, as well as the severity of your symptoms, referrals to specialists and/or further tests may be appropriate.

If there is concern about eye symptoms, for example, you may be referred to an ophthalmologist; if you have extreme dizziness or hearing loss with your attacks, a visit to an ear specialist and an audiologist might be in order. If attacks have worsened or are unusually severe, your doctor might want you to see a neurologist for a brain wave assessment (EEG) and/or a brain scan—either computerized tomography (CT) or magnetic resonance imaging (MRI).

I have had both an EEG and an MRI to investigate possible brain abnormalities, as well as an electronystagmography (ENG), administered by an audiologist to check for tumors on the cranial nerves. In my case, as is usual with most migraineurs, nothing alarming was found. None of these tests was painful, or even particularly unpleasant, although I did experience some dizziness and nausea after the audiological exam. Attaching and removing the required scalp sensors for the EEG is a messy process likely to disturb your hairdo, although no longer a painful one, as once it was. Some sufferers especially sensitive to flashing lights may develop a migraine attack after an EEG. If an MRI is ordered, your doctor may suggest a mild tranquilizer to relax you before the procedure. I experienced no difficulty having my MRI without medication, but can see the wisdom of the tranquilizer for anyone who is claustrophobic or otherwise anxious about lying still in a confined area for about 45 minutes. Relaxation or meditation techniques would serve you well during an MRI and might well take the place of the medication. Recently another aid has become available for patients who dislike feeling like a peanut in a shell—special glasses, called prism glasses, that actually allow seeing out of the tube-like device that surrounds you during the test. Your doctor or technician may be able to make those available on request. Just as a precaution, if you are required to submit to any of these specialized tests, consider asking someone to provide transportation in case you don't feel like driving afterward.

If you would like to become a well-informed patient before undergoing any of the tests suggested by your doctor, then you might want to seek information in the reference section of your public library about the purpose, preparation, procedure, and anticipated results of those specific tests. (Some helpful sources are mentioned at the end of the book.)

In most cases specialized tests will yield no noteworthy findings, leaving your doctor to diagnose your headaches on the basis of your clinical symptoms, that is, based on what you report having experienced and what he observes in you. Typically, severe headaches that come and go, and that are also accompanied by gastrointestinal symptoms and light sensitivity or other visual disturbances, are labeled as either common migraine or classic migraine.

Common migraine, which is experienced by over 80% of migraine sufferers, is considered as headache without clearcut warning symptoms, whereas the so-called classic variety has some sort of well-defined aura, either the familiar visual disturbances or some other sensory or neurological forewarnings. Many physicians seem to delight in attaching one or the other of these labels to migraines in spite of research findings indicating that the two labels may not represent distinct diagnostic categories. The line between common and classic migraine is hazy at best; frequently one person may suffer from both types of headaches at various times in her life or even alternately. Either variety may occur on one or both sides of the head.

Unfortunately there is no single diagnostic test to verify the presence of migraine. The disorder remains relatively mysterious and elusive, and in spite of extensive research and speculation, medical authorities still cannot identify with certainty the exact physical deficit(s) responsible for its excruciating misery. There is, then, still no universally accepted biological marker for migraine, like the blood sugar measurement used to help establish a diabetes diagnosis, for example. Thus, the diagnosis of migraine continues to be made primarily by a process of elimination. In summary, a physician assumes a patient has migraine largely on the basis of what the headache sufferer tells him, but only after ruling out the existence of other disorders that have similar symptoms.

After Diagnosis, Then What?

Assuming a migraine diagnosis has been made, your physician may be satisfied simply to send you on your way, or alternatively may offer you one of two types of medication: a migraine-abortive drug to be taken at the first sign of an attack in order to stave off the more painful symptoms; a migraine-preventing drug to be taken on a regular basis to forestall headaches; or both. Abortive medications may be considered appropriate if your attacks have distinct boundaries, that is, if they are discrete episodes, and if you consistently experience some warning signs well before the onset of the headache itself. Preventive remedies are apt to be offered if you experience more than two severe attacks per month or if symptoms are disabling and fail to respond to abortive medications. Some migraineurs may require a combination of the two approaches. (A detailed consideration of migraine medication is presented in Chapter 10.)

It is rather unlikely that your physician will offer you any in-depth lifestyle guidance, even though lifestyle factors are widely recognized as immediate triggers of migraines. The usual medical procedure is to take a brief patient history, perform a physical exam, order further testing if required and, lastly, prescribe medication, if such a prescription is both appropriate and desired by the migraineur. Seldom will the physician offer explanatory information regarding the nature of migraine, and seldom will the doctor devote much time to individualizing a prescribed drug to take account of either the patient's lifestyle or coexisting medical conditions. "Now, go take your pills and be happy" seems to be the prevailing philosophy. Never mind that even with the prescribed medication the headache sufferer may continue to suffer, although to a lesser degree if he or she is one of the lucky ones. For the less fortunate, unpleasant side effects may arise from the medication itself, only to compound the initial suffering.

Just because headache is a common complaint, neither doctor nor patient should assume that it's a simple one, either to diagnose or to treat. Quite the contrary. Unraveling the mystery of an individual's headache, especially pinpointing whether it is a disorder in and of itself, or a symptom of some underlying condition, requires both skill and persistence on the part of the physician. Following up on that diagnosis with an effective treatment calls for a careful, caring doctor, who will spend some time listening to the headache sufferer and tailoring the treatment to the patient's one-of-a-kind body and lifestyle. All of that represents a rather tall order in this age of 15-minute office visits. As the late Norman Cousins so aptly pointed out, insurance companies don't pay doctors for talking to their patients.

A Significant Partnership: *You and Your Doctor*

Because living with severe migraine is apt to be a lengthy, demanding, and frustrating experience, I believe that every sufferer deserves to work with a competent, cooperative, empathetic medical partner. My own notion of how such a partnership should function was inspired, at least partially, by the attitude and experiences of Norman Cousins in dealing with his two major illnesses. If you are not familiar with the way Cousins interacted with his physicians, informing himself and taking primary responsibility for his own wellness, you can learn about it by reading his own accounts in *Anatomy of an Illness* and *The Healing Heart*.

In a brochure sent to new members, the National Headache Foundation describes your greatest asset as a headache sufferer to be a "doctor who knows you and is willing to spend sufficient time to diagnose and treat your problems." I could not agree more.

Medical personnel themselves are finally beginning to realize that headache sufferers have traditionally received short shrift from the medical profession. We have been the victims of poor diagnosis, misunderstanding, and shotgun treatment. Although the situation might have begun to turn around, it still has a long way to go. An article in a recent German publication aptly refers to headache patients as "Medicine's Stepchildren," and a survey of 136 patients at the University of Minnesota Headache Clinic confirms a problem in this regard: Only 30% of chronic headache sufferers interviewed were totally satisfied with their treatment; 45% said their medication was ineffective; and about one third resented physicians' ignorance of headache disorders.

On the other hand, there is a small but growing group of physicians who apparently have devoted an extraordinary amount of time and effort to addressing chronic headache and associated symptoms. We can look to them for a model of the ideal migraine physician. Dr. Edda Hanington, well-known British clinician and researcher, and colleague Dr. Maurice Lessof outline physician responsibilities to include explaining why migraine attacks occur, working with a patient to consider all possible causes, and supervising a six-week trial diet. Education, emphasize Hanington and Lessof, is a critical but often-neglected element of treatment; these experts recommend that a physician give patients written material explaining the disorder. Dr. J. N. Blau, another renowned English migraine authority, agrees that it is the doctor's job to help a patient identify headache triggers. Blau, too, envisions a very comprehensive educational role for physicians. He sees their primary function as the ultimate restoration of the patients' ability to cope with their disorders independently.

My experiences with medical treatment fell far short of this ideal. For many years I was cheated of that most basic and important essential: an accurate diagnosis. Looking back, I realize it was the seventh physician I saw who finally diagnosed my symptoms accurately as common migraine. Based on the comedy of errors preceding this valid diagnosis, a comedy that spanned a decade and was frustrating and painful rather than funny, I have reached this conclusion: Some physicians, especially older ones, continue to consider only the classic migraine model when evaluating symptoms. I

can remember being asked whether I saw bright lights prior to my headaches and whether the pain was onesided. Negative replies to these questions shifted the focus to possible disorders of the gall bladder and inner ear.
The third family practitioner I consulted referred me to an ear specialist,
who in turn sent me on to an audiologist: these specialists misdiagnosed my
condition as Meniere's Syndrome, an inner ear affliction for which I was
offered little substantive help.

I now realize that I was probably experiencing what are called basilar
artery attacks, a term for a type of migraine marked by lightheadedness,
weakness, a temporary hearing deficit, and sometimes by ear noises called
tinnitus. All of these symptoms can be present in Meniere's Syndrome as
well, and so I can partially understand the reason for the confusion. Nevertheless I can't help blaming the misdiagnosis and my continuing misery on
my doctors' lack of knowledge. (The controversial relationship between
inner-ear disorders and migraine is addressed in Chapter 8.)

Finally, a bright young family practitioner recognized that I had migraine.
One primary difference between his approach and that of my previous doctors was the lengthy initial interview and history-taking session. I was
favorably impressed that he actually spent a significant amount of time
listening to me. His diagnosis was soon confirmed by a neurologist.

The Doctor's Role

In selecting a primary-care physician to treat your headaches, you might
ask yourself whether a particular doctor:

1. Gives you a view of the bigger picture, including what causes headaches and how lifestyle may impact them.
2. Listens when you talk.
3. Answers your questions and addresses your concerns.
4. Gives you credit for knowing something about your own body.
5. Seems to believe that you are in charge of your own wellness.
6. Explains options and asks preferences, as well as stating recommendations or simply giving orders.
7. Tells you how to take prescribed medications and what to expect from
   them; advises how to deal with any adverse reactions.
8. Explains test results and their significance.
9. Gives fair consideration to new medical information that you present.

It is highly unlikely that you will find a physician who meets all of these
criteria; but if yours falls far short, your headache might appreciate your
looking elsewhere. My own doctors are not perfect by these standards, but
at least they respect my intelligence.

The Patient's Role

Just as it will benefit you as a headache sufferer to locate a doctor with a special attitude, you'll likewise find it to your advantage to acquire an in-depth knowledge of your own condition. Be an informed medical consumer by becoming familiar with the migraine disorder and by keeping up to date with the latest diagnostic techniques and treatments. Unless your doctor really specializes in treating migraines, as few do outside of headache clinics, your physician may not be up on the latest research findings. If, however, that doctor is open-minded and more concerned about your welfare than his or her own ego, then state-of-the-art information will be welcomed. You may save yourself considerable misery by keeping abreast of the latest developments in the field and by tactfully informing your doctor about them. Some hints on how to gain this specialized knowledge are presented later in this chapter under the section "Other Resources."

Like me, you might have been socialized to believe that a doctor was the authority to whom you owed unquestioning obedience. Obviously I no longer accept that philosophy. Experience has taught me that the doctor does not always know what is best for me and, blasphemous though it may seem, may not even know what is best for my particular disorder from an objective medical point of view. I never automatically assume that the doctor knows best. If I feel a little shy about speaking out, I simply remind myself that my pain and my money are on the line. Then I usually find my voice.

Here are some appropriate patient responsibilities in this important working partnership:

1. Keep a detailed chronological record of headache symptoms and accompanying complaints; bring any changes to your doctor's attention even if they aren't requested.
2. Keep abreast of developments in the field of migraine diagnosis and treatment; inform or question the doctor regarding any significant discoveries.
3. Be willing to make appropriate lifestyle changes to improve your condition, rather than expecting the doctor magically to make everything better with drugs.
4. Ask for desired dietary, stress management, or other lifestyle guidance if it is not freely offered. (Even if the doctor does not feel personally qualified to provide this, perhaps you can be referred to someone who can.)
5. Inform your doctor about all other medicines taken, including vitamins and over-the-counter preparations, as well as about other known disorders, sensitivities, and allergies.
6. Ask about the purpose of, and procedure for, any recommended tests.

7. Tactfully remind your doctor whenever you believe something important has been overlooked.
8. If you accept a prescription, ask about directions and expected side effects.
9. Follow agreed-on decisions and directions, or else call or return to question them.

You have probably noticed that there is some overlap between the doctor's and patient's responsibilities as they are outlined here. Such double coverage is intentional. The theory is that since we all are human, we all will overlook important matters at least occasionally; this system of checks and balances should prevent anything significant from being neglected.

Dr. Dean Edell, medical journalist, offers the following tip concerning general patient/doctor communication. In a situation when a patient is unable to get a doctor to recommend a specific course of action or feels that the doctor is being less than totally candid about an opinion, Dr. Edell suggests posing the following question (to paraphrase his usual off-the-cuff style): Doc, what would you do if you or your spouse were in my situation? This query can elicit some very frank and helpful responses.

Headache Clinics: *State-of-the-Art Care*

At this writing, there are at least 28 clinics operating in the United States that offer specialized headache diagnosis and treatment. These clinics are geographically scattered so that almost every region is served by at least one of them.

Exceptions to this easy availability seem to be the Northwest and the Southeastern Seaboard regions. Those of you who live in the Northwest may find the closest clinic in northern California, and those who are in mid-Atlantic states may have to choose among Baltimore, MD, Richmond, VA, or the Pensacola or Orlando areas of Florida if you want this specialized care. A listing of these clinics is available from the National Headache Foundation or the American Council for Headache Education (addresses provided on page 10).

I have lived to regret not having visited one of these specialty clinics when my migraines first became severe. Had I done so, my chances of receiving an accurate diagnosis and more effective treatment early on probably would have been much better. It is my understanding that these clinics offer a more holistic approach to treatment than do most private physicians. Their medical staffs tend to be on the cutting edge, especially if they are research facilities, as many are.

Detailed information about fees, scheduling, and treatment options is available from the individual clinics; many, if not all of them, will gladly mail explanatory brochures as well. Some offer both in- and outpatient treatment. Your health insurance carrier can advise you what coverage it provides toward clinic treatment.

There is a headache clinic in Richmond, VA, about 70 miles from my home. The Center is staffed by neurologists and psychologists; an average waiting time for obtaining the first appointment is one week; the initial evaluation involves being seen by both a neurologist and a psychologist. This first visit takes between three and four hours and costs $385.00. Most health insurance providers pay between 50 and 80% of treatment costs. Many out-of-town patients are seen at the Richmond Center, and clinic personnel make every effort to arrange appointments to accommodate schedules and travel plans of clients. In order to avoid duplication, the Center requests forwarding of pertinent medical tests recently performed elsewhere.

Frankly, I do not know whether other headache clinics routinely include a personality evaluation by a psychologist as a part of their examination. That is something you might want to ask of a clinic you are considering. At one time I would have felt somewhat uncomfortable with the prospect of such an evaluation, thinking I might be told that I was emotionally unstable or that my headaches were "all in my head." Because I now know more about migraines, however, I view the situation differently. Realizing that the migraineur's body probably reacts less favorably to the biochemical effects of stress than does that of the average individual, I can see that we must compensate for our physical deficit by minimizing the harmful stress in our lives. The required adjustment seems to be somewhat akin to that undertaken by a visually handicapped person who must learn to rely less on her eyes and more on other senses.

If an individual cannot accomplish that daunting task of minimizing stress on her own, then working with a psychologist could be highly beneficial.

Other Resources

There are some valuable sources of assistance that allow headache sufferers to supplement personal medical care. Two national agencies conduct headache research, educate both the public and medical professionals, and provide a wide range of services to individual sufferers. These are the National Headache Foundation (originally formed in 1970 as the National Migraine Foundation) and the American Council for Headache Education, organized in 1990. Both organizations offer annual memberships for a modest fee; in return, individual members receive current research findings in the form of quarterly newsletters. Special brochures offering dietary and other lifestyle guidance are provided with initial membership. Publications dealing with topics of individual interest often are available to members on request. The National Headache Foundation has a toll-free telephone information service. Both organizations offer members a list of physicians (arranged by geographical area) who indicate an interest in treating headaches.

Here's where you may contact these national organizations:

National Headache Foundation (NHF)   American Council
5252 North Western Avenue   for Headache Education (ACHE)
Chicago, IL 60625   875 Kings Highway
1-800-843-2256, or   Suite 200
in Illinois, 1-800-523-8858   Woodbury, NJ 08096
                                         1-800-255-ACHE

Other valuable educational tools for those who wish to be well informed about current research are the medical journals *Headache* and *Cephalalgia* (a word of Greek and Latin origins, meaning head pain). You may locate these journals at some hospital and medical school libraries. Most such libraries are quite willing to allow nonmedical visitors to use publications on the premises. If these journals are not available in your area, or if you simply want personal copies, then you may purchase subscriptions from the following publishers:

Headache   *Cephalalgia*
PO Box 1897   Publications Expediting Inc.
Lawrence, KS   200 Meacham Ave.
66044-8897   Elmont, NY 11003 18

As of this writing, the yearly subscription cost for *Headache* is $95.00; *Cephalalgia,* which is published in Norway but provided in English for US readers, also costs $95.00 annually.

Other journals, many of which also will be available in your local medical libraries, publish significant headache studies from time to time as well. If you want to do in-depth research on migraine, your librarian can show you how to use the *Medical Index* and the publication *Books in Print* as sources that will direct you to pertinent articles and books. Then copies can be ordered conveniently and at a very reasonable cost through the inter-library loan system.

Another Resource: *Using the Remainder of This Book*

As the preface explains, this book is meant to assist you *only after* you have obtained personal medical care. If you have not already formed a satisfactory relationship with a physician and received a diagnosis for your headaches, please do so now.

But what if you do have a cooperative, respectful physician and yet do not feel completely confident with your diagnosis and/or treatment? In that case you may benefit from a second opinion, and you may be in a better position to deal with your doctors after reading the remainder of *Managing Your Migraine*, especially the first section of Chapter 8, which explores other conditions that are sometimes confused with migraine, and Chapter 10, which deals with medical treatments.

If you have accomplished both of these important steps—finding a satisfactory physician *and* receiving a confident diagnosis—then I offer both my congratulations and my empathy. I invite you to continue with Chapter 2, which briefly discusses the major difficulties and controversies among migraine researchers in recent years as well as the growing consensus about the nature of our disorder.

Chapter 2

Researchers Tackle a Tough One

Struggling with the Migraine Mystery

An Ancient Mystery Persists

For many centuries, headache sufferers and their physicians alike have wondered about what causes the strange sick-headache disorder we now call migraine. Apparently an ancient disease whose record is traceable into Babylonia and Egypt, migraine has long been depicted in popular and medical literature, as well as in art, as both fascinating and frustrating. Although much has been discovered about the malady over the centuries, particularly in the past few decades, certainly much remains to be learned, and even more to be completely understood.

In modern considerations, the disorder often is referred to as a "mystery," and terms such as "unraveling" are applied to attempts to understand it. Both literally and figuratively, progress in solving the mystery has been painfully slow. Rather than dwelling on the history of migraine, this chapter briefly considers recent developments in the battle to understand the disorder, while emphasizing the emerging medical consensus and some important practical implications of that knowledge.

Obstacles Yield to Progress

When one reads about migraine, one bit of information tends to jump off the page: The migraine attack is an extremely complex biochemical event involving dozens of changes in many parts of the body. The process often is called a "cascade." I like to think of it as a chain reaction, in which one small event sets off another, or even as an avalanche that starts small but gathers tremendous momentum as it moves. The biggest challenge for researchers, one still unmet, is to identify the initial chemical event in this reaction, the one that then activates all the others. Identifying that initial event has been difficult for a number of reasons.

During the past few decades, the migraine research arena has been an active one, but also one beset by numerous problems and disputes. Reading the history of that era, one is left with the impression that, to some extent, the participants have been spinning their wheels. Dr. Merton Sandler, a British expert, speaking to a group of the world's most dedicated migraine researchers gathered recently for a brainstorming session, pointed out with obvious frustration that migraine researchers continue to pose many of the same questions and wrestle with many of the same difficulties that occupied them some 40 years ago.

The casual reviewer may wonder whether scientific egos have interfered with medical progress as certain individuals grew entrenched in defense of their favorite theories of migraine causality. Thus, as researchers did verbal battle among themselves over the relative merits of various theories, our very real concerns as sufferers might well have taken a back seat at times. And, as is so often true in medicine, a desire for drug company profits seems to have controlled the research agenda.

In light of numerous and significant stumbling blocks, perhaps we should be both amazed and grateful for the substantial progress that has been made. These hurdles have included: the lack of a satisfactory animal model (further explained below); the enormity of personal egos; the deficiency of safe, morally acceptable techniques for viewing the human brain; and, for many years, even the very basic failure of researchers to agree on a definition of the disorder.

One avenue by which researchers try to pinpoint that all important precipitating event in the migraine cascade is by analyzing the various drugs that are effective against the disorder, looking for their common mode of action. Thus far, none has been found, but the trail is getting hot. In the last decade, the brain chemical serotonin has been attracting increasing attention. Many of the drugs found to be effective against migraine affect the level of this chemical in the brain. Recent success with the medication sumatriptan (sold in the United States as Imitrex), which works directly on this serotonin system, seems to confirm that researchers are on the right track.

It is gratifying to read about the research that is being conducted worldwide in order to try to unravel this ancient and especially stubborn mystery. As sufferers, our medical relationships tend to consist exclusively of contacts with harried practitioners, many of whom are uninformed or misinformed about migraine, and who may seem indifferent, unsympathetic, or even critical toward us as headache patients. I've certainly had my share of such disappointing contacts (as Chapter 1 describes), but delving into the workings of the research community gave me a completely different and much more optimistic perspective about the future of our disorder.

My emotional burden was immediately lightened somehow just by the knowledge that there are, at the very least, dozens of researchers worldwide whose primary focus is on understanding and relieving migraine. I was especially heartened by the work of British medical personnel, many of whom combine theoretical research and actual practice in a comprehensive and most impressive way. Western Europe and Scandinavia, too, are well represented by dedicated researchers. In Australia, Dr. James W. Lance and his colleagues deserve special mention for their innovative work in animal research.

Because headache is such a subjective experience, many researchers traditionally have bemoaned the fact that there is no good animal model for migraine. Because the presence of pain cannot be measured in an objective way and animals are unable to tell us whether or not they experience such pain, much less to rate it on a scale from one to ten, all researchers face obvious limitations in what they can learn through conventional laboratory methods. The Australian researchers, however, through painstaking experiments with monkeys and cats, have gained valuable insight into the nature of the disorder. By chemically and electrically stimulating the brains of such laboratory animals, Dr. Lance's teams are trying to determine exactly how central nervous system activity causes the blood vessel changes that occur in migraine.

In this country the work of Dr. Seymour Diamond, Chicago physician and researcher, has been especially impressive. Dr. Diamond not only directs a headache clinic devoted to both research and treatment, but also heads the National Headache Foundation, the first comprehensive source of information about migraine and other headaches for both the lay and medical communities. His persistent efforts are recognized as having been primarily responsible for the gradual, but significant, growth in knowledge about migraine as well as sensitivity to its sufferers. I am grateful for his insights into the relationship between migraine and depression and for his common sense acknowledgment of dietary triggers as immediate reasons for attacks, in spite of researchers' (including his own) inability to prove this dietary link conclusively in the lab.

Following in Dr. Diamond's footsteps, there is now emerging virtually a whole cadre of US practitioner–researchers based in headache treatment centers throughout the country. New voices are speaking out almost daily. Somebody cares! Particularly well known for conducting original research and getting the word out about the latest discoveries are Dr. N. T. Mathew of Houston; Dr. Joel Saper of Ann Arbor, Michigan; Dr. Seymour Solomon of Montefiore, New York; Dr. Lee Kudrow of Encino, California; Dr. K. M. A. Welsh of Detroit, Dr. Neil Raskin of San Francisco; Dr. John Graham (recently deceased) of the Boston area, and Dr. Stephen D. Silberstein of Philadelphia, to name only a few outstanding US migraine pioneers.

Particularly heartening is the holistic patient-centered approach of Drs. Alan Rapoport and Fred Sheftell, directors of the New England Center for Headache in Stamford, Connecticut, as outlined in their book *Headache Relief.* Now available in paperback, this book is a good investment—particularly valuable, as I see it, as a gift for an open-minded physician.

Current Medical Thinking: *Wolff Revisited*

The modern understanding of migraine is grounded in the work of Drs. Harold Wolff and Bronson Ray, colleagues at New York Hospital, who in the 1930s and 40s conducted the first systematic observations of physical changes occurring during headaches. Working with patients undergoing head surgery with only a local anesthetic, these researchers were able to confirm that long-suspected blood vessel changes were involved in the disorder—changes first suggested by an English physician several hundred years earlier. Later researchers, although not totally rejecting Wolff and Ray's theory of important blood vessel involvement in migraine, have looked beyond those obvious changes in blood flow toward the next level of causality. It may be helpful to think of this continuing investigation as similar to peeling back the layers of an onion.

Migraine detectives are now concentrating their efforts on mechanisms that regulate the tone of the blood vessels. These regulators, most now believe, are contained in the complex chemical network of the brain and central nervous system. To date, only a handful of these central nervous system chemicals, called neurotransmitters, actually have been identified, and many researchers believe that the ones known so far represent only the tip of the iceberg. Although these chemical interactions in the brain appear highly complex, our current understanding of them remains quite elementary.

So yes, although Wolff and Ray were correct in identifying blood vessel involvement in the migraine process, current researchers recognize that they probably were mistaken in concluding that those vascular changes were the basic cause of the disorder. It now seems probable that such changes in blood flow are instead secondary happenings. A defect in one or more of the neurotransmitter systems is suspected as the primary culprit. For the past decade, the chief suspects have been noradrenalin (also called norepinephrine), serotonin, and dopamine, all of which seem to play important roles in the process.

Particularly significant seems to be the balance between serotonin and noradrenalin. Serotonin affects a variety of bodily processes, including blood vessel activity; noradrenalin is a very important vascular regulator as well. When in proper balance, these two chemical messengers complement each other, leading to a smoothly functioning vascular system. One current theory holds that the vascular failure we call migraine results from a relative imbalance between these two neurotransmitters.

Other respected migraine detectives continue to hold that defective blood platelets, the tiny disk-like cells responsible for clotting, are actually the basic cause of migraine. Some significant differences in platelet makeup and activities have been found between migraineurs and nonmigraineurs. Most authorities believe, however, that these platelet differences, like the blood flow changes, are secondary to the migraine process rather than the primary cause of the disorder.

Agreement Grows

The remainder of this chapter focuses on the emerging consensus among researchers regarding the nature of our malady.

Children Can't Choose: The Genetic Basis of Migraine

Twin and other family studies conducted over the past few decades confirm what practitioners have long suspected, i.e., that the tendency toward migraine is inherited. Even though the responsible gene (or more likely genes) has not yet been identified, most researchers nevertheless feel confident in endorsing a genetic basis for the disorder. Somewhere between 70 and 90% of migraineurs (depending on which study one believes) report having close relatives who also suffer from severe headaches.

Australian authority Dr. James Lance explains a popular viewpoint on this matter of the genetics of migraine, pointing out that an inherited susceptibility is involved—what he calls a "migrainous threshold," rather than a dominant or recessive characteristic. Lance believes this threshold probably is determined by more than one gene and is therefore difficult to pinpoint. Furthermore, he compares it to the epileptic threshold, whereby one person may experience just one seizure during an entire lifetime, whereas another more susceptible individual may have regular episodes. Such an inherited threshold, Lance goes on to explain, leaves the migraineur vulnerable to internal fluctuations, such as hormone changes, for example, as well as to such other factors as environmental changes, fatigue, stress, and stimulating sensory experiences.

Detroit neurologist Dr. K. M. A. Welch endorses this same threshold theory of migraine, explaining that all individuals actually have the potential to experience an attack, but vary greatly regarding the weight of the factors required to trigger such an episode. Those of us who inherit a relatively low threshold, then, are at greatest risk for encountering triggers with sufficient power to set off many attacks during the course of our lives. To be absolutely accurate, if we accept this threshold theory, we should speak not in terms of black and white, that is, of migraineurs and nonmigraineurs, but rather of varying degrees of a basic human tendency. Indeed, if you talk to your female acquaintances, you may be surprised to discover how few of them have never experienced a severe headache accompanied either by light sensitivity, other visual distortions, or gastrointestinal symptoms—in other words, how few have never had a migraine.

Slippery Definition

Even formulating a basic definition of migraine on which most experts can agree has proved a challenge. Several slightly different ones exist—a fact that sometimes complicates diagnosis. In 1988, the International Headache Society (IHS) developed comprehensive criteria for all severe headache disorders, including several types of migraine. This should be helpful in conducting research, but some experts fear that these IHS definitions are too complicated and awkward to be used by the average physician.

Respected migraine researchers and practitioners, Drs. Seymour Solomon and Richard Lipton, propose a general migraine definition for everyday use—one that is being hailed by many as a workable model. According to these authorities, a headache that has *any two of the following four* qualities should be considered a migraine, *provided that* similar episodes have occurred previously and there is no sign of organic disease:

1. One-sided pain
2. Throbbing, at least part of the time
3. Nausea
4. Sensitivity to light or sound

It is important to recognize the following facts about migraines:

1. A headache is not required to be onesided in order to be classified as migraine—in fact, about one third of migraines are felt on both sides of the head.
2. A migraine need *not* be preceded by any sort of visual aura, that is, such visual distortions or manifestations as a limited field of vision, bright flashing lights, or zigzagged lines. As a matter of fact, fewer than 20% are signaled by any clear-cut warnings.

3. Although obvious vascular symptoms, such as throbbing, worsened by movement or coughing, often occur during at least part of the attack, these are not an essential part of the definition of migraine.

4. Duration can vary widely, from several hours to several days.

Distinct Categories Questioned: Toward a Continuum Theory

Classic Versus Common Migraine

Up until the past few years, many experts divided migraines into two distinct categories, i.e., classic migraine (CLM) and common migraine (COM), which were seen as stemming from somewhat different abnormalities in cranial blood flow. Now that researchers have begun to look beyond the vascular system into the central nervous system's regulatory mechanism for the ultimate cause of the malady, however, this division is being strongly challenged. In addition, although it is true that some sufferers consistently experience specific sensory warning signs, called an "aura" (most commonly a visual disturbance, although other sensory distortions often are involved) about 20–30 minutes before the onset of headache pain, the absence of such signs does *not* mean that a headache is *not* a migraine. Indeed, since it is known that some sufferers experience both varieties of migraine, either alternately or during different periods in their lives, common sense seems to confirm the unity of the disorder.

Tension Headache Versus Migraine

Likewise, the sharp division between tension headache and migraine is being closely re-examined. Until recently these two types of headache were seen as entirely different diagnostic categories, but the results of recent research call such a sharp distinction into question. Many experts now see headache as falling on a continuum closely tied to the relative supply of neurotransmitters. What was formerly called tension headache and thought to be caused by muscle tension or emotional stress, is now seen as a slightly different version of migraine, rather than an unrelated type of headache. Significantly, these so-called tension headaches seem to respond to many of the same medications that help migraines. Indeed, some authorities have come to believe that all headaches are merely variations of a common theme—all stemming from similar central nervous system malfunctions—differing only in degree rather than kind. One way to explain the change in the way in which different headaches are viewed is to say that rather than being thought of as distant cousins, all now are considered siblings.

Mixed Headache Syndrome

It has long been observed that as migraineurs age, the nature of their malady frequently changes significantly. Initially consisting of periodic,

ttacks separated by pain-free intervals, migraine often gradu-
es an illness in which major attacks grow less severe, but
milder headaches begin to intrude on the formerly pain-free periods. Previously this evolution puzzled doctors, who sometimes thought an entirely
different disorder was replacing the old migraine condition. More and more
experts now are coming to believe that such a change represents a normal
evolution in the disorder, and others suspect that common medications, specifically ergot preparations or even daily analgesics, may be responsible for
this altered course (which usually occurs ten years or more into the illness).
This later stage of the disorder is sometimes called "evolutive migraine,"
"mixed headache syndrome," or "chronic daily headache."

Because most migraineurs take ergot preparations or derivatives sometime during the course of their disease and many take daily pain medications
as well, it may be impossible to sort out what causes this change. The important point is to recognize that such an evolution is common and does not
represent the development of either tension or allergy headache.
Although these "new" headaches are milder than the accustomed ones, they
usually retain at least some of the vascular characteristics of the old
migraines. Rather than being a new type of headache, then, these milder
daily headaches are just migraine in a slightly different form (if we accept
the expert consensus)—and ones that respond well to traditional migraine
preventives, especially low-dose antidepressants.

Dietary Migraine

A significant portion of migraineurs have long realized that eating certain
foods makes them ill. In the 1920s and early 1930s, putting migraine
patients on very strict diets was standard medical practice even though there
was little, if any, scientific verification that such diets really were effective.
Gradually, traditional medicine began to lose interest in the dietary control
of migraine symptoms. Controlled experiments done in the past few decades
to try to define a possible relationship between diet and migraine have yielded
mixed findings, leaving a wide difference of opinion among medical professionals about this issue. It is probably safe to say that, outside of specialty headache clinics, you can expect requests for guidance on this aspect of treatment to
meet with either a great deal of indifference or a lack of knowledge.

In 1966, Dr. Edda Hanington, British physician and researcher (and herself a migraine sufferer), first noticed a striking similarity between the traditional migraine diet and a diet prescribed for people taking a new medication
for depression. That medication, called a monoamine oxidase inhibitor
(MAOI), had been introduced in 1962. It was widely heralded for its effectiveness in treating depression, but very soon a disturbing side effect

became evident. People taking this new drug began to have adverse reactions to some very common foods—reactions including a dramatic increase in blood pressure, accompanied by severe headache, nausea, sweating, and sometimes heart rhythm disturbances. Some of these people actually died as a result of ingesting an unfortunate combination—an effective new wonder drug and a perfectly ordinary food or beverage, such as aged cheese or red wine. Dr. Hanington and her coworkers soon noticed a striking similarity not only between the food avoidance lists drawn up for MAOI patients and the ones for migraineurs, but also between the symptoms of these two groups when they ate the offending foods.

From her observations about similar food reactions in migraineurs and MAOI patients, Dr. Hanington developed the amine avoidance theory of dietary migraine. She believes that dietary migraine sufferers are naturally deficient in monoamine oxidase, the same enzyme that is chemically blocked by the medication used by the depressed patients. In normal individuals, this naturally occurring enzyme breaks down amines, common nitrogen-containing substances in many ordinary foods. Dr. Hanington and some other researchers maintain that when certain dietary amines get into the bloodstream without having been chemically broken down, they cause specific blood platelet and blood vessel changes, triggering the process we call a migraine attack.

Although certainly not all experts accept the validity of this theory, it seems obvious to many that most common dietary triggers are high in these natural amines. Verifying this possible connection under controlled laboratory conditions has been difficult, however, and attempts to do so have yielded contradictory results. Scientists rely on a blood test to measure levels of monoamine oxidase in the body, but no one is sure that such a measurement gives an accurate picture of levels in the intestinal tract and liver, where the enzyme actually does its vital work.

Another group of British researchers has had better luck in establishing a link between dietary-induced migraine and a different enzyme deficiency. In controlled tests, Drs. Vivette Glover, Merton Sandler, and their colleagues have shown that migraine sufferers have lower than normal levels of an enzyme called PST. (The technical name for this body chemical is phenolsulfotransferase. Now you see the need for an abbreviation.) This enzyme is similar to MAO in that it breaks down dietary amines, but PST is also active against substances called phenolic flavonoids, which give the color to many common fruits and vegetables. Since there is no known safe way to correct either of these enzyme deficiencies, dietary migraineurs may choose to minimize symptoms by avoiding foods high in these substances (a topic addressed in Chapters 5 and 6).

The Future Agenda

Further research on exactly how the body uses serotonin is on the front burner in the wake of treatment successes with serotonin blockers like sumatriptan. Scientists already know that there are several types of serotonin receptors in the brain (cells to which that chemical binds or attaches), but they are working to better understand the function(s) of each kind and their specific roles in the migraine process.

Controlled trials are being conducted with other drugs as well. Some of the drugs under investigation as migraine preventives include the antiseizure medication valproic acid (sold as Depakene and Depakote), and a relatively new class of blood pressure medications called angiotensin-converting enzyme inhibitors (known as ACE inhibitors and sold as Capoten and Vasotec). Some researchers are excited about the new calcium channel blocker, flunarizine, already being used as a preventive in Europe and Canada.

Even the old familiar headache remedy aspirin is getting a new look—this time as a potentially important tool in headache prevention. The National Headache Foundation is studying 300 female sufferers, half of whom are taking one 325 mg aspirin tablet every other day, while the other half receive a look-alike drug. Results from this trial are expected very soon.

Another important and exciting area of investigation involves the use of new noninvasive methods for viewing or measuring brain function. These include two scans not yet in wide use, positron emission tomography (known as PET) and magnetoencephalography (MEG for short). Using these tools, researchers have already begun to measure brain blood flow as well as metabolic and neuronal function, both during and in between migraine attacks, in order to find out exactly how brain function affects migraine threshold.

The Big Picture: *The Status of the Mystery*

In summary, scientists have made impressive strides toward understanding migraine in spite of numerous significant obstacles. It is encouraging to realize that an energetic and dedicated group of medical researchers and practitioners around the world is actively battling our malady. A growing consensus holds a continuum theory of headache, replacing the previous sharp divisions between classic and common migraine and even between migraine and tension headache. Experts now tend to see all severe headaches as stemming from a similar brain-chemistry problem, probably involving some sort of imbalance or other malfunction among the neurotransmitters serotonin, noradrenalin, and/or dopamine and/or a defect in the receptor cells to which these chemicals bind. Blood vessel and blood platelet abnormalities now are viewed by most as secondary to the migraine process rather than as basic causes.

A strong genetic predisposition toward migraine is recognized, but even this is regarded as a matter of degree rather than an absolute—with many experts expressing the belief that, given the right circumstances, anyone is capable of experiencing a migraine attack. Some simply have much lower thresholds than others, thus requiring a lesser trigger exposure to set off such an episode.

Currently, any severe episodic headache accompanied by either nausea or a sensitivity to light or sound generally is classified as a migraine. Researchers realize that the disorder that begins with contained episodes frequently progresses to a stage in which vascular attacks alternate with milder daily headaches. Physicians who fail to keep abreast of the latest research may misdiagnose common migraine (migraine without a clear-cut aura), especially when it affects both sides of the head, because mistakenly they consider migraine to be onesided headache preceded by a specific visual aura—an incorrect and incomplete definition of the disorder. Likewise, poorly informed physicians are apt to mistake the nature of evolutive migraine, thus risking improper treatment.

Dietary migraine remains a matter of great confusion and controversy, with some experts holding that a deficiency in one or more enzymes is responsible for food-triggered symptoms.

As of this writing several new drugs are being tested either as migraine preventives or abortives.

Moving on to the Personal Level

Now that we all have a basic knowledge of the current understanding of migraine, we can move on to applying that understanding to our personal situations. Chapter 3 begins to explore some immediate concerns.

Chapter 3

Improving Our Odds

Triggers and Threshold-Setters

The Most Obvious Activators: *External Triggers*

This chapter is meant to assist you in identifying and avoiding personal triggers, primarily by discussing the way triggers work. If you have suffered from painful migraines for very long, then probably you've already made at least a mental note of some of the things that you believe precipitate your attacks. Such precipitators are called triggers. More than sixty of these triggers, including some widely diverse agents and experiences, have been identified by migraineurs, but relatively little research has been done to investigate exactly how these factors may work to bring about migraine, or to try to determine which ones might have been identified mistakenly by migraineurs because of honest confusion between coincidence and cause.

You might be aware that individual migraineurs have different triggers. And you might have noticed, as well, that your own response to these personal precipitators varies quite widely, even from one day to the next, not to mention from week-to-week or year-to-year. Regrettably, the reason for such varying responses remains clouded by the migraine "mystery," but many authorities have come to believe that such reaction variations are determined by certain conditions *within the body of the migraineur* at the time the external triggers are encountered. (A later section will consider that important topic.)

When Australian specialists George Selby and J. W. Lance asked 500 migraineurs about suspected triggers, 66% named stress, 47% cited glare, and 25% named certain common foods as sometimes precipitating their attacks. (Of course, each sufferer generally has numerous triggers, and these often change over time.) Triggers named in further surveys, either by sufferers or their physicians, are other very intense sensory experiences, such as strong odors, or even startling noises; dramatic changes in air pressure or other weather conditions; decreased oxygen supply; travel motion (especially that involving rapid head movement); a blow to the head or even tight head cover-

25

ings; inadequate, delayed, or missed meals; variations in sleep schedules; as well as the consumption of alcoholic beverages and certain preservatives.

In spite of the fact that both sufferers and their physicians tend to blame many attacks on stress, no controlled research conclusively forges the migraine–stress link. Indeed, many have come to question the conventional wisdom that stress is a common precipitator of attacks. Dr. Sheftell reports that his patients at the New England Center for Headaches cite alcohol, menstruation, and certain foods as their most frequent triggers. He and and I agree that the importance of stress as a migraine trigger may well have been exaggerated.

In the case of dietary triggers, chocolate, cheese, and citrus—sometimes referred to as the "three C's"—are the most frequently cited foods, although alcohol, especially red wine, is considered by many to be an even more potent offender. Controlled studies exploring the diet–migraine link have yielded conflicting results, and much disagreement remains among experts on this issue. However, research definitely pinpoints chocolate, red wine, and missing meals as dietary triggers in many individuals.

Understanding Triggers

Many experts believe that there must be a common pathway by which all of these, and possibly many other, precipitating factors work to cause the misery we call migraine, but, if so, it has not yet been identified. Certainly an overly sensitive central nervous system seems to be involved.

Dr. John Edmeads, renowned Canadian migraine authority, reinforced my desire to better understand triggers when he wrote that about 25% of migraineurs could achieve significant relief by learning to identify and shun triggers, and, as a result, could either avoid or minimize the need for medication. Or, looking at the other side of the coin, English expert Richard Peatfield stated that only about 70% of patients improve with medication, and very few see their attacks decrease by more than half. There seems to be a need, then, for a more comprehensive management strategy than merely taking drugs, and most experts agree that trigger avoidance is one of the most worthwhile steps in such a strategy.

In light of such a perspective, let's make an all-out effort to identify and minimize exposure to our personal triggers. The following principles will put us on the right path:

1. **Cumulative Nature of Triggers**. Dr. Edda Hanington convincingly presents and explains this theory in several of her articles. Other authorities agree, and my own experience and networking certainly confirm it. Once you grasp this basic concept of the cumulative nature of triggers, you will find zeroing in on your particular triggers much easier and less frus-

trating. For example, on Tuesday you may miss a meal without suffering any ill effect whatsoever, but on Saturday missing a meal will bring on a nasty attack. It is not enough, when evaluating the situation, to take into account only that one obvious trigger. You must also consider that the attack occurred on a weekend, when the letdown reflex comes into play, that you ate a chocolate bar the evening before, and slept in extra late that morning.

Viewed in this broader context, the missed meal takes on a different role. Apparently it was the straw that broke the camel's back—just enough of an additional weight when added to other potential triggers to cause an attack. On Tuesday, when other precipitating factors were not present, evidently the missed meal alone was not sufficient to lead to an attack.

2. **Trigger Lag Time**. The time between trigger exposure and the onset of attacks varies among individual sufferers as well as among different triggers at work within the same sufferer. In other words each sufferer has a slightly different timetable. In the case of dietary triggers, for example, researchers have established that a reaction can occur anywhere from three hours to 36 hours after eating offending foods, although most seem to happen within 12 hours.

For me, diet-related attacks begin about 18 hours after eating troublesome foods. Sulfites in foods, however, cause symptoms within just a few hours. In my case, acute emotional stress causes no immediate migraine symptoms, but I do experience the common letdown reflex after periods of prolonged stress or fatigue, at which time I seem to be more vulnerable to attacks. Certain environmental chemicals can cause headaches for me within a few minutes, as can exposure to heavy concentrations of dust. Every migraineur can benefit from becoming aware of her own personal reaction time to various triggers, and that awareness can be gained through the use of a migraine diary.

3. **Hormonal Triggers**. In female migraineurs, hormone fluctuations and the relative level of various hormones seem to be the most significant factors in determining trigger vulnerability. Women usually report the greatest vulnerability to attacks around the time of their menstrual periods and during early pregnancy, both times when estrogen levels are relatively low. Some studies show that in the case of dietary migraine, women are more sensitive to offending foods around the time of menstruation. Again at menopause, when another major hormone shift occurs, women often experience either an improvement or a worsening of symptoms. Oral contraceptives and certain forms of hormone replacement therapy make many women more vulnerable to attacks as well.

4. **Headache Diary**. This is the best tool an individual can use to pinpoint triggers. Keeping such a diary need not be a burdensome task or require a lifelong commitment. You may get significant help by keeping such a diary for about six weeks, noting symptoms by date, and rating their intensity on a scale from one to three, along with notes about any suspected preceding event, such as a heated argument, missed meal, beginning of vacation, extra coffee, new job, and so on. Female sufferers should include information about their menstrual cycle and/or hormone supplementation in their diary entries. (In Chapter 5, a detailed diet diary is suggested, but the ideal approach would be to combine dietary notes with these general entries.)

A plain notebook, kept in a convenient place where a pen or pencil is always available, can serve quite nicely as your diary. Better yet is a daybook or roomy appointment calendar in which days and dates are already marked and there is plenty of space for notes. Appendix A outlines a sample format for diary entries. You may begin your diary-keeping now, or you may decide to wait until you read the next six chapters. By the time you explore the information presented in that portion of the book, you will be much better able to pinpoint your own triggers and threshold-setters. Over time, and possibly with the help of your doctor or an empathetic friend, you are likely to recognize a pattern that explains many, if not all, of your attacks.

Those who experience daily headache are probably the least likely to benefit from keeping a diary. Even so, such record keeping may be enlightening if more severe attacks are interspersed with the milder daily ones, as is often the case. (Such sufferers first need to determine whether or not they are abusing drugs—such as caffeine, nicotine, ergot, butalbital, or even aspirin and acetaminophen [Tylenol]—that may be causing their daily pain.)

My own use of a headache diary helped me to identify and assume control over one of my important environmental triggers—house dust. As far back as I can remember, I have sneezed when exposed to dust. I had always assumed that this slightly annoying reaction stemmed from a mild allergy and then dismissed it as unimportant. That picture changed dramatically after my migraine attacks began. What had been of no consequence before could then usher in days of pure misery.

Initially, however, the role of dust exposure was not all that clear. I had to do some basic detective work. At first, with the help of my diary, I simply noticed that on days when I performed dusting and vacuuming chores, I often experienced attacks by late afternoon or early evening. Because of something I had read, I suspected strained neck muscles might play a part. Then one day while emptying my vacuum cleaner bag, I accidentally exposed myself to a giant whiff of dust. Dramatic migraine symptoms began within less than fifteen minutes. It was only after a repeat performance—that is, another accidental dust exposure followed by almost immediate symptoms—that I was confident I had found my trigger. Use of an efficient dust mask (one with chipped coconut shells as a filter) eliminated the worst of my housecleaning symptoms. Although wearing the mask is uncomfortable, that discomfort is insignificant compared to my previous migraine pain. (To be extra safe at vulnerable times, I take half a dose of a garden-variety antihistamine about 30 minutes before starting my chores.)

A Difficult but Worthwhile Battle

If you are getting the feeling that trigger identification is rather complicated, no doubt you're right. Currently, the bottom-line process remains one of trial and error—a scary prospect, when one thinks of the painful consequences of those inevitable errors, but don't despair. Persistent use of your diary—noting the principles stated above—eventually will lead to less pain and more control over your life.

More Fundamental Causes: Threshold-Setters

Everyone is familiar with the saying about "the straw that broke the camel's back," a metaphor I have already called into use to help explain the cumulative nature of triggers. Carrying the analogy one step further, this same metaphor also can be useful in illustrating one of the reasons that a particular trigger is more powerful at one time than another.

Imagine that the camel's humane and thoughtful owner purchases a back-saving saddle for his pack animal. After the camel dons its protective saddle, the animal is then able carry a much heavier load without suffering any ill effects. If the owner, however, in great haste to get to market one morning, carelessly fails to strap on the saddle, then that very same load may prove too much for the poor beast. The saddle re-sets the animal's load threshold, as it were, just as many migraine authorities believe certain hormone levels, other medical conditions, drugs, lifestyle choices, and chronically stressful situations can re-set our headache thresholds—either up or down. Remember the camel as we explore these various factors and try to see how our reactions to various triggers are influenced by the type of saddle we're wearing at the time.

My own experience may serve as an illustration. I was 35 years old when I suffered my first full-fledged migraine attack. (As I mentioned in the preface, I had experienced some mild episodes as a child and teenager that I failed to recognize as migraine.) I recall that December day vividly—the day of my first severe attack. I had been wrapping Christmas gifts and had eaten one of my favorite lunches, a peanut butter sandwich and an orange. I also had been using cleaning solvent to remove wax from my young daughter's favorite slacks. Sometime late that afternoon I was hit with severe lightheadedness and dizziness, soon followed by a feeling of fullness in the head and ears, and then, several hours later, by nausea and a painful headache totally unlike any headache I had ever had.

What was different about me on that December day in 1975 that caused such bizarre symptoms? Certainly my genetic makeup, any central nervous system deficit I might have inherited, was basically the same as it had been during the previous 35 years, and I hardly think my environment was entirely unique to that day, either. Obviously something had changed, however, and I believe that "something" was what British migraine authority Dr. J. N. Blau calls "internal disposition," exactly the same idea that we have been referring to as the migraine threshold. Something had changed within me to lower that threshold, and because of that internal change, certain external factors—those triggers we've been talking about—were suddenly able to make me desperately ill.

What could have happened in that "fatal" 35th year that resulted in such a dramatic lowering of my threshold? Our knowledge of migraine, sad to say, may be too elementary to allow us to pinpoint the exact cause or causes, but I consider the following happenings as prime candidates: my changing hormone status associated with impending menopause; chronic, low-level exposure to a toxic chemical, i.e., improperly applied chlordane, which had been used as a termite treatment in our home several times in the years immediately preceding the attack; and/or a period of prolonged family stress that I was experiencing during that phase of my life.

My research suggests that any one of these factors could have been responsible for lowering my threshold. Certainly the three of them might well have worked together to make me vulnerable to migraines, allowing free rein to an inherited susceptibility. At any rate, as a 35-year old woman, I suddenly "gained" migraines, one might say—perhaps a peculiar way to describe the onset of a highly undesirable experience.

"Losing" and "Gaining" Migraine

To look at another common scenario, this process often works in reverse. Just as often as someone gains migraine, another person will at some time in her life lose her migraines for no readily apparent reason. After all, I had lost my mild childhood migraines for more than 15 years. I'd venture a guess that some of you may have had such an experience as well. Women often report losing their migraines during the last two trimesters of pregnancy.

Frequently, too (although not always, by any means), older women who might have suffered attacks all their lives happily note losing them after menopause. In some of these instances, no matter how great the exposure to former triggers, no headache results.

Several of my acquaintances have related losing childhood migraines after becoming adults. I can't help wondering about the role of dietary triggers in such cases. Often adults dramatically reduce their consumption of migraine-provoking foods such as chocolate (especially in the form of chocolate milk), peanut butter, pizza, and hot dogs, all of which tend to be everyday fare for many children. In my own case, sometime in late adolescence I developed an actual allergy to chocolate (resulting in swelling and hives), after which I very rarely ate it. That dietary omission might have contributed to the changing migraine status that I experienced at about that time in my life.

One friend noted this pattern, which in some ways is similar to mine: moderate childhood attacks, but a noticeable decrease in both number and severity on entering adulthood; a gradual increase as she approached menopause; and still further worsening with the beginning of hormone replacement therapy after a hysterectomy. The woman herself was not aware that these seemingly mysterious changes in the intensity of her symptoms over the course of a lifetime were probably not just happenstance occurrences. Each of these changes, whether it be a very dramatic loss or gain, or a somewhat more subtle waxing or waning, probably has a specific cause or causes, which, at least in some cases, can be identified and modified.

As was mentioned earlier, in women hormone changes are the most likely causes of changes in migraine activity. In both male and female sufferers, changes in lifestyle, health, and stress levels are closely associated with changes in the level of migraine symptoms, as is taking certain medications.

It was Dr. J. N. Blau whose work really stimulated my interest in this topic of the changing migraine threshold. In a very interesting study, Blau looked at life changes suspected by 52 sufferers as responsible for their loss of migraines. Participants were recruited by Blau via a newsletter published by the British Migraine Association; all reported experiencing at least a two-year remission from attacks, and the average period of remission was eight years. Blau himself pointed out that the genetic backgrounds of these individuals obviously did not change. He went on to reason that trigger exposure probably continued at much the same level as before and concluded that a change in the sufferers' internal settings somehow weakened formerly powerful triggering agents so that these factors no longer were able to set off attacks.

Reasons for these remissions, as identified by the migraineurs themselves, were broken down as follows: eleven cited decreased stress levels; ten cited menopause; five, dietary changes; one, hormone treatment; four, blood pressure medication; three, surgery (two had hysterectomy and one an operation for peritonitis, an infection of the abdominal wall); one, diabetes medication; one, acupuncture; one, chiropractic treatment; four, nonspecific "physical" changes; and one, "drinking a half pint water in the morning"! The remaining ten subjects did not even venture a guess to explain their "losses."

As Blau himself was careful to emphasize, one cannot necessarily accept the explanations given by the migraineurs themselves as the real reasons for their remissions. Nevertheless, it is certainly obvious that remission from migraine does occur, and it is probably not unreasonable at least to try to identify the reason or reasons for it. I myself want to thank Blau for initiating this innovative and valuable area of investigation. I hope that he or other researchers will continue to pursue it.

In the meantime we can pursue it together by looking into several possible areas that may affect our migraine susceptibility. Our genetic predisposition is a given: Obviously we have no control over that. Our opportunity for relief lies in the areas of raising our threshold and avoiding triggers. The remaining chapters examine different aspects of these efforts.

Better Control Through Careful Evaluation

If you have noticed a significant change in either the frequency or intensity of your headaches at some time during the course of your disorder, then your migraine threshold might have changed. The self-evaluation form provided in Appendix B may help you begin to pinpoint the responsible factors. This evaluation can be helpful in the long run regardless of whether or not you have experienced a recent change in your symptoms. The more you know about how various factors in your life affect your headaches, the more control you can assume over them.

If your headaches have worsened recently, please consult your physician before going on. Otherwise proceed with the self-assessment before reading further. Once you become more aware of some of the factors that may underlie your problem, Chapters 4 through 9, which discuss common triggers and threshold-setters in detail, should allow you to move into the next phase—getting a handle on them.

The Big Picture: *Triggers and Threshold-Setters at a Glance*

1. Triggers merely represent the immediate reason for migraine attacks in susceptible people rather than the most basic cause, which is thought to involve one or more inherited defects.

2. The power of triggers to lead to attacks varies significantly even in the same person, depending on the internal disposition or threshold-setting of that individual at the time of exposure.
3. In women, hormone status is believed to be the most powerful threshold-setter. Other important factors in all sufferers include chronic stress, various physical disorders, and medications.

Chapter 4

How Lifestyle Contributes

Live Right and Thrive

A Matter of Control: *Schedule Regularity*

Some migraine sufferers feel discouraged when they learn that their heredity predisposes them to headaches. In fact, if we are honest, many migraineurs will probably admit to occasional bleak feelings of hopelessness and loss of control; I certainly have experienced many such low times. However, although those feelings are based in the reality that there is no simple cure or perfect control for migraine as I write this, our present situation is actually far from bleak. I believe that we are quite capable of reestablishing control over our lives if we are serious about applying our present knowledge and pooling our existing resources.

Let's begin this process of regaining control right now by examining those facets of our personal lifestyles that have been shown to influence migraine significantly and that are already under our control. In each case, the experts are in general agreement about the ways these factors enter into the migraine equation. The first is schedule regularity. Research studies show, and many sufferers confirm, that maintaining regular eating and sleeping patterns is of utmost importance in any migraine management program.

Grazing on the Clock and Other Blood Sugar Issues

Specific research recommendations are that we go no longer than five waking hours and 12–13 hours overnight without eating. That translates into three squares a day on a fairly regular schedule, because failing to eat either enough food or the right kinds of food at mealtime may cause problems for migraineurs just as readily as actually missing a meal. For example, British authority Dr. J. N. Blau suggests that a breakfast consisting only of a bowl of cornflakes might well constitute an inadequate meal for many migraineurs. A better choice would be a whole grain cereal (no added bran or malt) with extra wheat germ, accompanied by a whole piece of fruit. Such a breakfast probably would get most of us through the morning because it contains sufficient amounts of both protein and fiber, two substances that tend to stabilize blood sugar levels. (*See* Chapter 6 for further dietary suggestions.)

In the same vein, when a meal is delayed, a snack high in both protein and fiber should be eaten. A glass of low-fat (1/2%) milk and half an apple would be a good choice (unless you have a known allergy or intolerance to one of these foods), offering a combination with plenty of staying power. Between meals, it's best to avoid caffeine and quickly metabolized carbohydrates, like candy or fruit juice, because both tend to send your blood sugar on a rather nasty roller-coaster ride.

If you have an unpredictable schedule, dietary requirements must be attended to before the need arises. Stash some appropriate snacks at work or school, for example, or at least have a contingency plan for snacking. Realizing that your dinner hour has passed as you sit in the middle of a meeting does no good; you will benefit only if you took precautions by having a snack beforehand, or at least prepared a ready reason to excuse yourself briefly to get that thermos of milk from your desk. If special events require you to retire late, a bedtime snack may be in order. Then it's advisable to get up no more than an hour later than usual the next morning so that meals can be approximately on schedule.

Experts disagree among themselves about whether or not migraineurs who experience attacks as a result of late or missed meals are actually suffering from low blood sugar, technically called hypoglycemia. Since arbitrary levels are used to define this blood sugar disorder, it is probably not really important whether or not a technically defined hypoglycemia exists, and having sufferers submit to the six-hour blood sugar laboratory measurement (glucose tolerance test) to determine this relatively arbitrary matter doesn't make much sense. (This test, which can be quite uncomfortable, is not considered highly accurate.) It might be worth your while, however, to request a fasting blood sugar measurement the next time you have blood work done. That very basic test, which is both easy and inexpensive, could alert you to a previously unrecognized problem.

Even if you don't test out as being hypoglycemic, however, delayed or missed meals may still trigger attacks. Picking up on this trigger can be tricky because there may be a time-lag between the missed meal and the start of the attack. Some researchers believe that low blood sugar causes a release of vasoconstrictive chemicals; if that theory is correct, then symptoms may not appear until after these chemicals wear off. With a little astute observation, aided by your headache diary, you can be the best judge of your own reaction in such situations.

If you have no established meal schedule, however, you might easily miss such a connection. In that case, it would be wise to set up a trial run of at least six weeks to determine whether migraine symptoms improve. During that period, adhere to the migraine guidelines by eating at least every five or six daytime hours and within 12–13 hours overnight. If you feel noticeably hungry before those time limits, then have an appropriate snack.

Certain medications and hormone supplements can wreak havoc with blood sugar levels. If you notice either a general worsening of your migraines or some specific symptoms of low blood sugar (weakness, nervousness, trembling, excessive perspiration, and confusion) after beginning a particular medication or supplement, check the product insert leaflet available from your pharmacist or the *Physicians' Desk Reference* (PDR) in your public library. If your medication/supplement is known to affect blood sugar, then consult your doctor about the cost–benefit ratio, with an eye toward either reducing dosage, switching to a medication without that undesirable effect, or simply eliminating the medication entirely.

In the event of elective surgery, the lengthy period of presurgical fasting can present a nasty problem for migraineurs whose attacks are triggered by missing meals or by abrupt caffeine withdrawal. Your surgeon should be told if this problem is anticipated. You and he may want to consider an intravenous feeding before the operation to forestall such an attack.

Exercising strenuously or for lengthy periods when you are noticeably hungry, or shortly before meals, risks migraine symptoms because exercise is known to lower blood sugar temporarily. Therefore, it's wise for sufferers to schedule their exercise at other times.

Female migraineurs may notice that blood sugar problems first appear or intensify during their premenstrual phase each month. Research shows that many women actually need more calories at that time, so that regular, well-balanced meals become even more important then. It's essential to be consistent in minimizing sugar and caffeine while increasing the intake of protein and complex carbohydrates. This is a particularly critical phase for women because it is both a time of increased vulnerability to attacks and a time when potentially troublesome food cravings raise their ugly heads. Chocolate is a common craving that spells trouble for many migraineurs. Eating regular, satisfying meals becomes an absolute must. Most people are less likely to give in to cravings if they are comfortably full of more healthful foods.

If you are weight conscious and find all of this talk about frequent eating somewhat disconcerting, not to worry. Eating more is not necessarily required, just eating smarter. For some people that means eating the same amount of food over a longer period of time. Many busy people fall into the rut of postponing substantial eating until late in the day when they have the leisure to prepare and enjoy a good meal. They may honestly fail to feel hungry earlier, may simply ignore bodily signals, or even grab something quick and often sugary, like a donut, to quiet their growling stomachs. Migraineurs who want to feel their best will find ways to change that pattern, even if they must get up half an hour earlier to eat a real breakfast and pack a substantial lunch.

On the other hand, severely restrictive weight-loss regimens, crash diets *per se*, are probably not compatible—at least for most of us—with migraine prevention. The limited calories called for simply do not allow for maintaining even blood sugar levels.

Giving blood causes a temporary drop in blood sugar that could trigger your migraine symptoms. Although few need fear participating in this noble activity, there are some precautions to bear in mind: It's probably wise to avoid donating when you're having symptoms or when you're in a particularly vulnerable phase (just before or during menstruation, for women, for example, or during a very stressful time); if you're on an aspirin or NSAID regimen, it might be advisable to discontinue it two weeks prior to the donation, especially if you've noticed any excessive bleeding after minor cuts; and it's probably a good idea to eat a full meal no more than two hours before the actual donation (allow about 30 minutes for the interview that precedes it); taking your own beverage and/or snack along may be a good idea as well (those provided are often heavy on citrus, caffeine, and chocolate); and, lastly, plan a relatively easy day in case symptoms develop afterward. I give blood on a regular basis, but I *do* pick my times carefully. The worst post-donation symptoms I've ever experienced were minor weakness and lightheadedness, lasting no more than an hour.

A Personal Blood Sugar Battle

It always has been quite apparent, even before I began to experience recognizable migraine attacks, that I felt much better when eating sensibly. Going back to my preteen years, I have clear memories of feeling irritable, disoriented, dizzy, and lightheaded whenever meals were either inadequate or delayed. It didn't take long for me to catch on and make special efforts to eat properly. In middle age, when my first severe migraine attacks began, I would sometimes experience mild headaches associated with hunger, but never thought a severe attack was caused by lack of food alone. More commonly, I still react to prolonged hunger with irritability and inability to concentrate. Then after eating, I frequently experience nausea and continued fatigue, instead of snapping back as one might expect. On one recent occasion my main meal was unduly delayed because of a reservation mixup at a restaurant, and although I didn't notice any immediate problems, I did experience mild headache symptoms all the following day.

Low-fat milk literally has been my salvation when it comes to maintaining even blood sugar levels. Not only is this beverage high in protein—the quality that makes it a good blood sugar regulator—but it is also both portable and widely available. As a bonus, of course, it is an excellent source of calcium and other beneficial nutrients as well—all for a moderately low calorie cost. (Of course drinking milk is not appropriate for those suffering either a lactose intolerance or an actual allergy to the beverage. These topics are discussed in Chapter 6.) As mentioned above, I find that I get better results when I eat something high in fiber along with the milk—a piece of fruit, a couple of plain rice cakes, or a handful of Triscuits, for example. Indeed, studies investigating blood sugar control among diabetics confirm that fiber plays a vital role in maintaining even levels.

I have noticed an increased problem with low blood sugar since I began taking Prozac, an antidepressant/migraine preventive, and using an estrogen skin-patch as part of my migraine prevention program. The problem has been minimized, but not entirely eliminated, by reducing the doses of both drugs. After carefully weighing my options, I decided to tolerate this side effect because both medications provide substantial migraine relief and I am able to work around the blood sugar problem by eating small, frequent, high quality meals and snacks.

ZZZs by the Book

Sleep is the other major scheduling concern. Whether this is actually an independent risk factor or just another facet of the food or stress component has not yet been sorted out. It has been observed, however, that we migraineurs feel better when we sleep on a regular basis—that is, when we retire and arise at approximately the same time every day. On weekends and holidays it is probably best to sleep no more than one hour past your normal wakeup time. If you feel like extra rest later in the day, a nap of no more than a hour should cause no problem as long as it does not delay meal times unduly.

The ideal strategy is to take reasonable precautions to avoid becoming overly tired. Learn to divide demanding jobs into manageable tasks and to take short breaks during the course of your day. It was amazing to me to discover how refreshing even two minutes of deep breathing or gentle muscle stretching could be. A ten-minute walk away from the desk or soaking in a warm tub at home can be nearly miraculous. If your body is really tired, just a 20-minute nap can work wonders. Here's where a relaxation tape can come in handy by helping you unwind so that you can really benefit from these brief respites. Let me assure the work-oriented among you that any one of these activities may actually increase a day's production; looking at the situation from that perspective keeps the conscientious worker from labeling breaks as luxuries or time-wasters.

Stress: *Trigger and/or Result*

The other essential lifestyle strategy is stress reduction. Some migraineurs notice an immediate triggering effect from extreme emotional upsets—a particularly heated argument with a significant other, for example. Others, like me, do not experience that type of immediate feedback from our bodies, but suffer instead from the more common "letdown" reaction—symptoms appearing only after the stressful event has passed. Whichever the pattern, immediate or delayed, most experts agree that long-term exposure to high levels of stress can increase the incidence of migraines in susceptible persons. Such an exposure seems to be a threshold-lowering factor.

On the other hand, migraine experts are moving away from the traditional view that stress is a common migraine precipitant. Whereas many sufferers and their physicians continue to blame attacks on stress, specialists more frequently note that attacks are triggered by other factors—such things as alcohol, menstruation, and certain foods. Sometimes those who continue to link stress to migraine define the term "stress" very broadly—including not only emotional upset, as we might expect, but also various physical stressors, such as hunger and fatigue.

The term "stress" indeed can be a very broad one—so broad, in fact, that at times it becomes almost meaningless. Different people use this word in very different ways—sometimes referring to the external events and experiences (more properly called stressors) that seem to trigger stressful reactions, and sometimes referring to a person's physical and mental/emotional responses to such external experiences.

No one knows for sure exactly how stress acts to worsen migraine symptoms, but experts assume that complex biochemical changes are involved. Most of you are probably familiar with the fight or flight syndrome. The adrenaline and related stimulating chemicals, known as vasoconstrictors, produced by our bodies when we feel threatened by real or perceived danger may be at the core of the migraine–stress connection. Some experts believe that migraines develop in predisposed individuals when these stimulant chemicals begin to decrease and blood vessels start to expand again—a theory that fails to explain why some sufferers experience immediate ill effects in stressful situations. It does, however, address the more common response—that is, the delayed or letdown reaction. Only later, after the excitement subsides and the sufferer starts to relax does the migraine attack typically begin. How many of you have experienced postexam attacks, weekend attacks, or vacation attacks?

Most often we think of stress as a negative experience, but it may be important to note that even the excitement associated with pleasant changes is stressful when it requires us to adapt. These positive experiences, too, cause biochemical changes that may upset the migraineur's body, but since positive stressors are primarily pleasurable, few of us would want to curtail them. For that reason this chapter concentrates on dealing with negative experiences and responses. Even when coping with pleasant excitement, however, many intense people might well benefit from learning to slow down.

Migraine Personality: Fact or Fiction?

You probably have heard about the stereotypically anxious migraine sufferer—one who is an intense perfectionist. It is only natural to feel somewhat defensive when we hear ourselves and other sufferers described in this way. Let me assure you that the jury is still out on this issue of the migraine personality—whether sufferers typically display certain personality traits. Although physicians have observed a common roster of traits in many of their migraine patients, these qualities may reflect a chicken or egg situation. Does the patient's anxiety cause the headache, or is it the reverse? Are the most anxious patients also the most likely to visit their doctors frequently?

I have to level with you that there is indeed some recent evidence suggesting a link between anxiety and migraine. Even if further research confirms such a connection, however, we should not interpret it to mean that we cause our attacks because we allow ourselves to become too worked up over something. Such an interpretation would be a simplistic half-truth, at best. If there is a constitutional anxiety–migraine link, it appears that the same biochemical predisposition leads to both conditions. The only point about which there is near universal agreement thus far is that the migraineur's body does not handle the biochemical results of stress as well as the nonmigraineur's. Therefore it seems prudent that we try to keep our lives on a relatively even keel and to minimize stress as much as possible. Ah, yes, but much easier said than done, you protest, and of course you are absolutely right.

Declawing the Tiger: Stress Reduction

As a counselor who sometimes instructs clients in stress-management techniques, I will resist the temptation to reinvent the wheel. There are many excellent stress-reduction resources available in public libraries and health or bookstores. Here are a few books you may find helpful:

*The Assertive Woman** by Phelps and Austin, 1985.
Happily Ever After by Helmerling, 1986 (for couples).
Is It Worth Dying For? by Eliot and Breo, 1984.
Learned Optimism (especially Chapter 10, "Health," and Part III, "Change from Pessimism to Optimism") by Seligman, 1991.
The Relaxation Response by Benson and Klipper, 1976.
*The Superwoman Syndrome** by Shaevitz, 1984.
Treating Type A Behavior and Your Heart by Friedman and Ulmer, 1984.
Woulda, Coulda, Shoulda by Freeman and Dewolf, 1989.
Your Perfect Right by Alberti and Emmons, 1974.

For those who would rather listen than read, many audio and video tapes are available on this subject. Chances are good that your local public library offers some. One very short and straightforward audio featuring media physician Dr. Art Ulene is called simply *How to Relieve the Effects of Stress.*

Now let's look briefly at some practical ways to minimize negative emotional stress. I like to use a three-pronged approach to stress reduction. Before we can put any antistress strategies to work for us, however, we must first get in touch with our individual stress reactions. Some of us may clench our jaws or grind our teeth when upset, for example, or may find ourselves drumming our fingers when we become impatient; or, quite commonly, our reactions will occur on the emotional rather than the physical level. We may become unmotivated or depressed, losing interest in ordinarily pleasurable experiences and becoming generally passive toward life for a time. Once we recognize our own particular signals—whatever they may be—then we can work backward from those and take a look at the precipitating events, with an eye toward either:

1. Changing the situation or escaping from it.
2. Changing the way we view or interpret the situation.
3. Simply deciding to accept the situation while devising ways to work out any negative feelings associated with it.

Think of some stressful situation in your life and try to figure out which of these approaches looks most promising. Quite possibly some combination of two or even all three will work better than any one alone. Actually, as you will see in the example below, in real life these approaches do not fall into the separate categories outlined here; however, when planning a strategy, you may find it helpful to think of them as independent options.

*Valuable for men as well as women.

For example, if you feel resentful about required overtime on the job, you might try to change the situation by scheduling a private talk with your supervisor about it (approach #1). Even if that effort fails, you may feel better just for having made it (touching on approach #3). Then you could try a little self-talk to try to change your perspective: Remind yourself how fortunate you are to have such a good job and that the overtime will probably let up at the end of the season (approach #2). Third, you might invest some of your extra pay to hire a household helper, thus reducing your after-hour chores and increasing your leisure time (approach #3). If, after all of these efforts to decrease your resentment, you still find the situation intolerable, you might return to approach #1, taking a much more radical course: You could quit your job and escape the unpleasant situation entirely. Of course, before taking such a drastic action, you would want to take a hard look at your financial situation and other possible employment opportunities.

This general approach stems from cognitive-behavioral psychology, a school of thought formalized by Dr. Aaron T. Beck of the University of Pennsylvania. Dr. Beck and other cognitive psychologists emphasize the point that how we choose to look at a situation greatly determines how that situation affects us. Obviously this strategy does not offer a quick fix for your stress-related problems; it is merely a framework that may help you more clearly see and evaluate possible options in various situations. My counseling clients seem to have applied this framework beneficially in some areas of their lives.

Negative Feelings: We'd Rather Ignore Them

Accepting a situation while figuring out how to deal with negative feelings is a very important stress-management technique, one that many people seem to neglect. If you tend to bottle up such feelings as anger, frustration, and disappointment—trying to minimize them or pretend they don't really exist—you instead may be creating a great deal of internal stress. Consider buying a simple notebook and using it as a journal. (This could be a section of your headache diary, but you'll need plenty of room for writing.) Select a couple of weeks when you anticipate a little lull in your life, and at a convenient time each evening, try to remember experiences about which you felt stressed or negative during the day. Then write about them in a simple but descriptive way, emphasizing your exact feelings at the time. Write as if you were talking to yourself—you are—using any sort of grammar, sentence structure, and vocabulary that leaves you at ease. If you feel more comfortable literally talking to yourself, then get out a tape recorder and address those same negative feelings orally. Once you practice this skill and begin to feel as comfortable airing your feelings as sweeping them under the rug, you can begin turning to your journal only when you're aware that something is beginning to gnaw away at you (in the scenario of forced overtime described above, for example.)

Another helpful technique for dealing with negative feelings is to write a letter to the person with whom you're upset. You need not plan to send it; simply write a letter directed to the person with whom you are angry, frustrated, resentful, disappointed, or whatever, stating exactly how you feel toward him or her—and why you feel that way. Then put the letter away until you cool off. In a few days, re-read what you've written, and think about whether you actually want to send it. You might want to ask the opinion of a trusted friend before you make a final decision, for an objective person may help you better sort out the probable consequences of such an action. Regardless of whether you send the letter, the very act of having written it (and of having read it aloud to another person) will help you deal with, and possibly take the self-destructive edge off, your negative feelings.

Some more comprehensive ways to deal with negative feelings: If you find that you consistently have trouble saying no and later feel frustration because of this inability, consider taking an assertiveness training course. And if you tend to fly off the handle, saying things you later regret, consider an anger management course. Both of these courses are frequently offered at very minimal cost by hospitals, public or private health agencies, or community colleges, or check with your local United Way Agency for a possible source.

Talking It Over: What the Doctor Ordered

Just having a safe place to discuss problems and vent feelings is a great stress reducer. Is there a personal-growth group in your community that you might feel comfortable joining? If you are a survivor of an abusive or traumatic childhood, look for a support group such as ALANON or Adult Children of Alcoholics (ACOA). ALANON, a spinoff from Alcoholics Anonymous (AA), is available without charge in nearly every community and specializes in assistance for anyone who has had, or currently suffers, a troublesome relationship with an alcoholic—whether parent, spouse, child, or good friend. The ACOA groups are specifically for adult children of alcoholics; some of them are free self-help groups much like AA and ALANON, whereas others are for-profit ventures led by professional counselors.

Because there is a very wide range of support groups available in most communities these days, there is a good chance of locating one that meets your needs. If you are uncertain what might be available where you live, hospitals are usually good sources for such information. Frequently churches and synagogues sponsor such groups or allow them to meet on the premises. If you find that much of your stress revolves around dealing with your migraine disorder, contact the American Council for Headache Education (address provided in Chapter 1) for guidelines on how to organize a headache support group. In spite of the popularity of medically related support groups, those dealing with chronic headache still seem to be relatively scarce.

We All Know How to Relax: Or Do We?

It seems as if the ability to relax should come naturally, but it doesn't always work that way. If you find yourself feeling unpleasantly tense or geared up when you'd like to gear down, perhaps it's time to investigate learning some formal relaxation skills. One of the easiest and least expensive ways to acquire such skills is by using relaxation tapes available through your library, health store, bookstore, or the National Headache Foundation. Find one you like and use it for about 20 minutes a day, or see the text in Appendix C to create your own tape, either by recording it yourself or getting a friend with a pleasant voice to do it for you. (The sample included is a short version just to give you a feel for what relaxation skills are all about.) If you prefer, you can buy a tape for no more than $15.00. The National Headache Foundation (address in Chapter 1) has a couple of general ones. In addition to promoting an ability to unwind, these tapes are great as sleeping aids if you have an insomnia problem or simply need a little help after being awakened by a nighttime headache. *See* Chapter 10 for a discussion on biofeedback, a closely related technique that requires medical instruction and supervision.

Both of these antistress strategies—general relaxation techniques (often promoting progressive muscle relaxation) and biofeedback—have been shown in controlled research studies to be effective migraine preventives and abortives. The idea is to use the tape(s) for a while as a practice aid, at least until the relaxation response becomes automatic. After a few months of daily practice, many people are then able to set the tape aside, and continue to reinforce the skills on their own. Research shows, however, that regular practice is necessary to obtain full benefit from these relaxation or biofeedback exercises. Experts speculate that such practice actually stimulates the production of antistress substances counteracting, at least in part, the vasoconstrictive chemicals produced during stressful experiences.

I have tried a number of slightly different approaches to relaxation, ultimately preferring to work with self-hypnosis tapes. At first I was reluctant to try anything labeled hypnosis until I realized that this form of relaxation is just that—relaxation—rather than some magical mumbo-jumbo used by one person to control another. When I first began using the tapes, I was a little surprised to discover that no awareness of present reality was lost; I simply became better able to push aside unwanted thoughts for a time.

My favorite commercial hypnosis tapes are *Introduction to Self-Hypnosis* by James Zinger and *Two Exercises in Hypnosis* by Dr. Jean Holroyd (*See* Suggested Reading/Listening at the end of this book for ordering information). Each tape lasts about 20 minutes. I have to admit that I do not use them every day, as I probably should to achieve maximum benefit; but I do enjoy them at least several times a week—usually when I'm feeling unpleasantly tense or excited, or when I feel a headache coming on.

For simple fatigue, these relaxation procedures are even better than a longer nap because there is no residual drowsiness. I love the way I feel after practicing my relaxation skills. It's that same cozy feeling that we all enjoy when we first begin to wake up in the morning and know that we are free to sleep in if we choose—a pleasantly warm and heavy body accompanied by a mind free from distractions and able to do some really creative thinking, or to do absolutely nothing at all. But more to the point, I have some modest success in using the tapes to minimize the mild symptoms that I currently experience.

One well-known relaxation technique with which I am personally not familiar is transcendental meditation (the form of relaxation that was so popular in the 60s and probably still has a number of adherents); from what I've read, I believe it would produce a satisfactory antimigraine response. On the other hand, I am very wary of the so-called subliminal tapes now being sold as relaxation tools; I have seen no evidence that these are legitimate, and, frankly, I consider them mere gimmicks.

I urge you to master some type of relaxation skill—whether it be the general variety, self-hypnosis, meditation, or medically supervised biofeedback. Any one of these will likely prove a very versatile tool, serving you in many ways as you struggle to manage your illness.

But I've saved the best for last. Possibly the two most potent stress busters involve (a) achieving at least one close, supportive relationship and (b) engaging in a regular aerobic exercise program.

Creating an Oasis in the Desert

If you are involved in a close relationship that produces a significant amount of stress rather than support, a serious investment of time and money may be called for. Assuming that this is an ongoing situation that you are not prepared to leave, and that you and your companion are unable to fix alone, then it may be time to seek professional help. If stress is a trigger, then continuing to subject yourself to chronic stress in such a relationship may be asking for headache problems.

Ideally this primary relationship should provide a safe oasis for escaping life's other stressors. After all, most jobs are at least somewhat stressful, and if you come home to another predominantly stressful situation at the end of the work day, you are depriving yourself of any real opportunity to let your hair down. If your relationship fails to provide such a haven, consider looking for a clinical psychologist, a licensed counselor, or a social worker who specializes in couples' work. Ask around for someone with experience and a good reputation for achieving practical results. The stigma of seeking such help is fading fast, and many medical insurance polices provide at least partial coverage. Your counselor or insurance representative can advise you about the details of your particular policy. If one partner suffers anxiety because of problems in the relationship—as could certainly be claimed for a migraineur—then the policy will probably cover couples' treatment, even if the language of the policy specifically disallows marital counseling.

In 1989 my husband and I decided to seek couples' counseling in an attempt to improve our 28-year relationship. For two years, we worked with a licensed clinical social worker on a weekly or semiweekly basis. Yes, it was expensive and time-consuming and also emotionally painful, but, most importantly, the results more than justified all the costs. I have never thought that stress was a significant trigger for my migraines, and improving this important relationship confirmed that belief, but we are both much happier people as a result of that work, and, as you might expect, we get along much better as a couple. That's worth a lot. You probably have a feel for whether relationship stress is a headache trigger in your particular case and can decide on that basis whether such counseling would be a worthwhile anti-migraine strategy for you.

Generating Natural Pain Relief

After you have been given the green light by your doctor, consider beginning a regular aerobic exercise program. Long recognized as an effective stress fighter, aerobic exercise may offer special benefits to migraineurs because of the natural antipain substances it produces in the brain.

For maximum benefit from an exercise program, you need to keep moving your arms or legs (or both, if you're already very fit) continuously for 20–30 minutes—but not necessarily at a rapid pace, especially in the beginning. If you are just setting out on such a program, most experts would advise starting slowly, gradually increasing both time and intensity, and backing off at the first sign of pain or discomfort. (Starting gradually, and slowly building activity levels may be even more important for migraineurs than for less headache-prone individuals.)

If you are just starting to exercise, the most important considerations seem to be picking activities you enjoy, alternating them occasionally, varying the locale, and exercising with a companion at least part of the time. Walking, biking, and swimming are usually good choices. Research confirms that paying attention to these factors helps assure sticking to a regimen over the long haul. Forcing yourself into some boring activity, and then trying to hang on by the skin of your teeth, is not the wise way to go.

Neither is it a good idea for exercise-minded migraineurs to wear tight-fitting helmets or headbands, popular in some sports, or to schedule exercise sessions when hungry or shortly before mealtime. Either can bring on a headache—the tight headgear because it seems to sensitize unstable blood vessels and the latter because exercise temporarily lowers blood sugar. When exercising in brightly lighted locales, migraineurs would be wise to shield their eyes with an efficient pair of glasses, either colored or clear ones providing full ultraviolet (UV) protection. A brimmed hat or cap may help as well. In addition, experts warn that migraineurs traveling to high altitudes should not attempt strenuous exercise for several days, until their bodies have had time to adjust to the less dense atmosphere.

The growing consensus seems to be that many migraineurs would benefit from a regular aerobic program, at least in the long run. A study done at a Canadian university and described in the January, 1992 issue of the medical journal *Headache,* found that 11 migraineurs who participated in a six-week aerobic exercise program experienced a significant decrease in pain. Indeed, an earlier issue of the same journal cited a case study in which an aerobics instructor reports that she can stave off an attack through strenuous exercise performed when subtle warning symptoms first appear. Others, however, recognize that strenuous exercise causes or worsens their symptoms. Of course, you are the best judge of your own personal response. It may well be that how your migraine symptoms respond to exercise depends on your current fitness level. Obviously the aerobic instructor mentioned above has achieved a very high level of fitness.

I get my aerobic exercise in approximately 45-minute increments, enjoying walks with an interesting friend three days a week; our schedule is preset in early morning for our mutual convenience. The rest of the time I bike, sometimes alone, but more often with my recently retired husband. We are fairly flexible with the schedule of our outings, but early morning stints still seem to leave me feeling best. In the little really bad weather we experience in balmy coastal Virginia—most often the excessive heat and humidity of the summer rather than cold winter miseries—I drive my car to the comfort of the nearest mall where conditions are always right. (Mall walking is becoming quite popular all over the country, especially among the senior crowd who sometimes form clubs, meeting for coffee and conversation after their walks.) In all, I usually succeed in putting in six sessions a week and continue to find them pleasurable as well as beneficial to my sense of physical and emotional well-being.

At times I have been able to "work off" symptoms by walking briskly *very early* in an attack, although I now approach such walks with caution since I have become faint on several occasions. When I'm experiencing symptoms, I make it a rule never to go out alone. Sometimes, with the mild episodes I now experience, improvement can be obtained from relatively gentle floor exercises. Several acquaintances have also reported that aerobic exercise brings them considerable migraine relief, both in reducing the number of attacks experienced as well as in staving off symptoms once an attack begins.

Be Sure It's the Right Tiger

As a reader of Norman Cousins and other proponents of the mind–body connection, I am quick to affirm that stress can trigger migraines, as traditional wisdom holds. Even so, my informed hunch is that this explanation of the origin of attacks has been significantly exaggerated, especially in the case of female sufferers. It seems to be easy for doctors to blame symptoms on stress or even hysteria, and then to dismiss them as inconsequential. Many angry women relate having had this experience.

Probably the biggest danger in so hastily blaming stress is that other—possibly more easily addressed—triggers are overlooked. Several examples come to mind. A sufferer invariably experiences severe attacks after plane trips. If stress is blamed, no one will ever figure out that the nitrite and MSG-laden airline lunch was really to blame. (Changing air pressure is also a likely cause of flight-related symptoms.) Another migraineur frequently has attacks after visits to the dentist—not all visits, but whenever cavities are filled. She assumes that her anxiety triggers these attacks, whereas the chief suspect should probably be the powerful vasoconstrictor contained in the dental anesthetic. So don't be overly eager to stalk the stress tiger.

In addition, keep in mind that this mind–body connection is a two-way street, in spite of the fact that the popular media commonly emphasizes how the mind affects the body. Don't forget the other lane—in our case not only can stress trigger migraine miseries, but frequent, severe pain can lead either to stress or to depression, or both. (For a discussion of this complex interrelationship and some ways of dealing with the body–mind avenue, *see* Chapter 11.)

I took great pains to declaw all my major life stressors, and I haven't regretted it for even one minute. On the other hand, neither can I honestly say that my migraine symptoms improved as a result of my less stressful life.

Slow But Sure

Pick just one of these antistress strategies that looks potentially helpful to you. Consider it thoughtfully, planning how you might best put it into practice; then discuss your approach with a trusted friend. At that point you will be in a good position to start implementing the strategy. Work on each appropriate area for four to six weeks, making it part of your routine, before embarking on another area of potential change. The idea here is to keep good intentions from going the way of most New Year's resolutions. If you are an impatient person like me, this suggestion may cause you some frustration, but in the long run, you will likely achieve greater success—and in this case, possibly less headache pain—by taking the slow approach.

Smoking: *An Obvious Culprit*

Because nicotine is known to be a powerful vasoconstrictor as well as a potent source of both carbon monoxide and formaldehyde, migraineurs who are serious about regaining control must stop smoking or using tobacco in any form. Period.

Surveys that contrast migraine symptoms in sufferers—first while they continue to smoke and then after they quit—strongly support the the notion that nicotine worsens both the frequency and the severity of attacks. A recent controlled research study also suggests that smoking worsens migraines.

Smokers' knowledge that they may die of a heart attack, stroke, or lung cancer in 30 years only infrequently provides them sufficient reason to quit. If it were otherwise, there would be no smokers, because those risks are solidly documented. Other types of consequences seem better at motivating smokers to end a bad habit. Some female smokers become motivated to quit when they are shown pictures of other women with smoking-induced wrinkles around their mouths. Vanity is apparently a stronger motivator than long-term health concerns. But what about immediate comfort and well-being? Doesn't that count for something? Having a migraine attack is a much more immediate and dramatic result of smoking than are those mouth wrinkles.

When British migraine specialist Dr. E. C. Grant surveyed 336 migraineurs in a London headache clinic in the 1970s, she confirmed a dramatic link between smoking and migraine. Her smoking patients had significantly more frequent and more severe symptoms than the nonsmokers; the smokers, logically enough, were therefore more likely to seek medical treatment for their attacks. But the most compelling information uncovered by Dr. Grant was that, on cessation, the former puffers experienced a tenfold drop in the number of their migraine attacks.

I know two apparently enthusiastic smokers who express extreme anger with their doctors' apparent inability to cure their migraine disorders. Isn't something very amiss with that logic? I can only agree with the prudent doctor who refuses to prescribe potentially dangerous medication to such patients, who, because of lifestyle choices, are very unlikely to benefit significantly from it anyway.

Probably the most serious long-term health risk for smoking migraineurs is stroke—and that constitutes a very real danger. A 1991 study addressing stroke risk in migraine sufferers estimates that even a nonsmoking sufferer has, on average, twice the stroke potential of a nonmigraineur. (Please realize that the risk is still low, just greater, for the average migraineur without other risk factors.) Common sense tells us that since smoking is also widely recognized as a leading stroke inducer, an individual who suffers migraine and still smokes must be quite a gambler.

Help: Appropriate and Available

Modern medicine has come to realize that nicotine is a highly addictive drug, just as powerful as heroin or crack cocaine in its ability to enchain its victim. If you want to stop smoking, it certainly is appropriate to seek assistance. Consider contacting the local chapter of the American Lung Association or the American Cancer Society for tips or referrals to a reputable treatment program. If those agencies themselves do not offer free or low-cost cessation programs, then in most cases they can refer to other local nonprofit groups who do. Some hospitals, for example, offer inexpensive or even free treatment.

In some communities where nonprofit treatment is not available, fee-charging programs may be the only option. Even if treatment fees amount to several hundred dollars, that still won't compare with even the patient portion of a major medical evaluation if your headaches worsen and you are required to have sophisticated testing (not to mention the cost of other medical problems down the road). Investing in a smoking-cessation program, if there are no free ones in your community, really makes sense from both a financial and a health point of view. Be sure to check with your employer, because more companies are now paying for employee treatment, or at least offering a financial reward for successful completion. Some even provide in-house smoking-cessation treatment.

Your doctor may be able to help here as well. If you have followed the route outlined above and continue to be troubled by a nicotine addiction, there are several medical options. In the recent past, some smokers have been helped over the hump by using nicotine gum; the currently available nicotine patches reportedly are easier, more pleasant, and more effective than gum because they release the chemical more evenly. The usual protocol is to wear the patch for two or three months, but in slowly decreasing strengths, thus avoiding the very unpleasant jolt of sudden chemical withdrawal. Because the very newest patch, Nicotrol, is removed at night, it is less likely to cause bothersome side effects than earlier versions.

Further medical aids include a low dose of clonidine (sold as Catapres), a medication normally given in higher doses for cardiovascular problems. This drug has demonstrated effectiveness as a smoking cessation tool. Alternatively, believe it or not, an antidepressant might be in order. Recent studies show that smokers who experience difficulty shaking the habit often are suffering from a mild form of depression and have been relying on the nicotine to boost their low moods. Antidepressant drugs have a good track record in assisting those individuals and may be particularly appropriate for smoking migraineurs. Since experts now recognize depressive tendencies in a significant portion of the migraine population, and antidepressants have proven to be effective migraine preventives whether or not depression is present, a trial run on a low-dose antidepressant regimen makes a lot of sense. The same medication that can help a person give up nicotine also can improve migraine symptoms in other ways.

Please don't be reluctant to use one or more of these aids if you have been unable to quit smoking, or, more commonly, to "stay quit" on your own. Be aware that even the most determined-to-quit smoker often does not succeed in quitting permanently until she tries several times; so if you don't make it the first time, don't give up—just keep trying. I, myself, am a former smoker who didn't succeed in staying quit until after three serious tries. At the time I was first struggling to quit many years ago, I wasn't smart enough to know about various available sources of help, and, indeed, there weren't as many of them at that time anyway. Please don't hesitate to take advantage of the many different resources that are available to "quitters" today. Your body will love you if you succeed in winning this important battle.

Special Environmental Influences

Since we know that people commonly gain or lose their migraines, it only makes sense to look to an individual's surroundings for possible headache influences. Our own everyday choices, at least to some extent, determine those surroundings—making them an area of personal control.

Computer Terminals/Video Games

Whether required by our work or simply indulged in as hobbies, video devices have become a regular feature of 20th century life. Since they are a source of bright and fast moving visual stimulation, these devices also can act as migraine triggers. Here are some important points to remember as you indulge:

1. Lighting in the room should be adequate but not glaring, and most importantly, no bright light should be shining directly into your eyes or reflecting off your video screen; for example, avoid facing a sunny window and place any lamps several yards off to the side of the monitor rather than directly behind or in front of it (these glare-avoidance tips also apply to television viewing). Commercial filters available in your computer supply store are very helpful in decreasing glare from your terminals.
2. Short frequent breaks should be taken as you work or play; get up and do some simple stretching exercises every 20–30 minutes if you feel tense, or simply walk into the kitchen and get a glass of water once an hour; children would be better served by alternating physical activity with the passive video games rather than making the latter an all-afternoon marathon.

Noxious Fumes and Odors

Many migraineurs report being particularly sensitive to certain fumes or odors—a heightened sensitivity that is recognized as part of a more general hyperreactivity to sensory stimuli of various sorts. In fact, any one of the senses can be involved in migraine, either acting as a trigger or exhibiting distortion before or during an attack. Commonly, however, we tend to hear about visual triggers and distortions to the neglect of the others. Although experts certainly recognize that olfactory experiences (what we smell) can trigger attacks, this area seems to have been neglected in the headache literature.

If you find any odor particularly offensive, it makes sense to minimize or avoid exposure. If you are sure that specific odors trigger or worsen symptoms, then heroic avoidance efforts may well be worthwhile. Some potentially troublesome chemical sources along with situations to be avoided are listed in the table on the following page.

Of course our greatest sources of exposure to these unpleasant, and for some of us dangerous, odors are our homes and workplaces. It is hoped that these places represent our greatest areas of control as well. I personally am

Chemical	Situation
Perfume/hairspray/mousse	Personal use; confined areas (cars/elevators) in presence of heavy users
Permanent wave solutions	Personal use; beauty salon employment
Car exhaust	Peak-traffic driving/outdoor exercise; use of tunnels
Fresh paint	Enclosed areas for up to 6 months (heaviest concentration usually dissipates within 1 month)
Waxes/varnishes	Personal application/presence in enclosed area within several days of use
Formaldehyde	Exposure to new fabric or carpet, recently decorated buildings; carpet stores/fabric stores/clothing stores, especially at the beginning of the season; particle-board furniture; foam urea insulation (RVs/mobile homes/new car interiors are particularly troublesome sources of this chemical)
Cigaret smoke	Any heavy concentration, especially in poorly ventilated areas
Outgassing plastics	New appliances that heat (dishwashers/hood hair dryers/computers)

very sensitive to odors. Now that I am taking a preventive medication, however, this sensitivity has decreased significantly. Allow me to share with you some of the measures I have taken in both my home and office to avoid these offending smells.

At home, I avoid buying furniture or gadgets made from particle-board or plywood, looking instead for used pieces of solid wood or unfinished pine products. In some cases metal items would do nicely, but expense tends to be prohibitive. Cotton or wool carpets with jute pads or backing are less offensive than synthetics. When painting, I have only one interior room done at any given time and then only in early spring or fall when I can ventilate daily for the next month. Usually I spread out the newspaper for a few hours before reading it because I find the fresh ink bothersome. For the first two years after purchasing a new dishwasher, I used the heat-dry cycle only when weather permitted opening windows; and I bought a used computer to minimize outgassing. During the period when my attacks were at their worst, I gave up my hard-hat hair dryer along with permanent waves, hairspray, and mousse. I now use hair spray sparingly in my open garage with towels covering my face and shoulders. (Some beauty-supply houses sell face shields to lessen spray exposure.) In this same vein, I find the newer cool perms less bothersome than the heat-activated ones.

I avoid most strong household cleaning products—having rediscovered the wonders of simple liquid detergents, borax, vinegar, and baking soda for such tasks as washing windows, scrubbing bathrooms, or keeping drains clear. (Aerosol products are especially troublesome because of the obvious difficulty in containing them.) Lots of outside air is absolutely essential on the rare occasions when I use a stronger product. I launder new garments before wearing and new fabric before cutting or sewing. Garments from the dry cleaners must be aired for several days before I wear them.

At work, I make an issue of others' smoking when they do not follow regulations. I avoid new or recently decorated buildings if at all possible. I ask maintenance people to refrain from using sprays and other offensive cleaning products in my presence, and I avoid being near wet duplicating machines or laser printers. Even felt-tipped pens, in a poorly ventilated area, are items to be avoided. Generally when ventilation seems poor, I open a window.

Formaldehyde is so prevalent in our world that I'm sure total avoidance would be impossible. Still, in addition to aggravating migraines, this chemical is recognized as a definite animal carcinogen and a possible human one. Even the conservative American Lung Association cites it as at least potentially harmful and recommends minimizing exposure. That organization warns that formaldehyde exposure can cause headaches, dizziness, and nausea, as well as asthma attacks in susceptible people. Exposure to high levels of this chemical can result in some individuals' developing permanent sensitivity to even low levels of the substance, according to the Association.

That agency recommends purchasing special low formaldehyde-emitting pressed wood products for indoor use, as well as covering objectionable sources with appropriate coatings and/or sealers. (One expert advises that three coats of either oil-based paint or polyurethane will decrease outgassing significantly; this should be done outside and allowed to dry thoroughly before bringing the item back in.) The Lung Association points out that high temperature and humidity speed formaldehyde release. Cigaret smoke, in addition to its other negatives, also contains a significant amount of formaldehyde, according to this same source.

Interestingly, NASA researchers recently completed studies showing the effectiveness of several common house plants in removing this risky chemical from the air; they recommend the spider plant and golden pathos for formaldehyde absorption. Another possible help for the chemically sensitive who are forced to remain in formaldehyde-ridden areas is a mineral called zeolite, which purportedly absorbs certain chemical gases, including formaldehyde. Zeolite is marketed under the trade name NonScents by Krueger Enterprises of Iowa City, Iowa 52240 (Route 5, Box 148). (A wholesale chemical company might prove to be a less expensive source for the substance.)

Motor Home, a magazine devoted to the interests of recreational vehicle owners, reports that a significant number of such travelers attribute unpleasant symptoms—including headache, dizziness, and rashes—to formaldehyde exposure from their vehicles. Since the mid-1980s most manufacturers have been using low-emission pressed wood or even solid wood products for walls and cabinetry in such vehicles, but carpet continues to constitute a significant source of formaldehyde and other fumes; and in such close quarters, almost any source is a reason for concern for the sensitive individual.

The National Institute of Health (NIH) warns that vascular headache can result from exposure to insecticides, carbon tetrachloride (a cleaning compound), and lead, encountered in paint, batteries, or lead-glazed pottery—particularly dishes manufactured in other countries, where standards are less exacting. Art materials, too, are common headache triggers, according to this same source, which cites exposure to turpentine, spray adhesives, rubber cement, and certain ink as especially troublesome.

In our ever more environmentally conscious world, new products frequently are introduced into the marketplace claiming to be less toxic than previous versions. I have noticed such claims for indoor house paint (Glidden makes a latex one, only in shades of white, that they claim contains no volatile organic compounds and is odor-free) and carpets (manufacturers add a green tag). Some skepticism may be in order about the safety of such products until convincing studies are released or usage establishes a track record. In fact, some recent studies of the new "green" carpets show that although formaldehyde may have been reduced, other harmful chemicals actually have increased. The Environmental Protection Agency (EPA) continues to test carpets in an attempt the determine exactly which chemical(s) pose the greatest health risk. The EPA refuses to say which substances may be suspect, but when they refurbished their own headquarters in 1988 after workers complained of chemical-related symptoms, only carpet without 4-phenylcyclohexene (4-PC) was purchased. Some researchers believe that 4-PC, which appears in most carpet backing, causes headaches, nausea, and eye and throat irritation.

Multiple Chemical Sensitivity: A Related Disorder?

I have often wondered whether or not there is a link between the chemical sensitivities shown by some migraineurs and those exhibited by the victims of the disorder known as multiple chemical sensitivity (MCS), or environmental illness (EI). For the unfamiliar, these terms describe a syndrome that is characterized primarily by chemical hypersensitivity. Sufferers usually trace the beginning of their symptoms back to an acute or chronic exposure to some insecticide or other toxic substance, but after that experience, the smallest exposure to a whole host of chemicals can trigger or intensify symptoms. MCS can affect only one body system or several. An afflicted individual might experience symptoms related only to the respiratory or gastrointestinal tract, for example, or to both of those systems as well as the cardiovascular network.

I believe that some chemically sensitive migraineurs may fit the diagnostic criteria for this disorder as well. In fact, I myself was actually told I had MCS even before I was diagnosed with migraine. I first began to experience severe migraine attacks after chronic exposure to the pesticide chlordane that was misapplied to our home by a poorly trained termite-control technician. He sprayed this highly toxic substance underneath and all around our house on several different occasions after termite damage had been sighted. At the time our chief concern was protecting the structural soundness of our residence against feared termite damage, and we naively trusted the operator to apply the chemical safely. By far the heaviest application, as well as the last, was made in 1982 (when federal regulation finally required a much safer application method than spraying). For years afterward, we could smell a strong odor whenever the house was closed up and heated. Not fully realizing the danger to which we were being exposed, we probably failed to compensate by providing adequate ventilation. During the years following those misapplications, my troublesome migraine symptoms first appeared and gradually worsened. Only after many years of misery did I began to suspect and investigate the possible role of chlordane in my predicament.

Frighteningly little information is available on the health effects of low-level pesticide exposure. Most research has been directed toward evaluating the hazards of massive contamination. However, one preliminary study done in 1987 by researchers from the University of Illinois School of Public Health in Chicago suggests a possible link between low-level chlordane exposure and migraine occurrence. When this study investigated the health status of 261 people residing in 85 households previously treated with chlordane for termite control, the incidence of migraine correlated highly with the measured indoor air levels of the chemical.

The authors of the Chicago study caution that this correlation, significant though it appears, does not demonstrate a cause-and-effect relationship between chlordane exposure and migraine. The findings certainly raised my antenna, however. Unfortunately, I have found no other studies investigating this possible chlordane–migraine connection, but I find it fascinating to note that closely related pesticides have been shown to inhibit enzyme production after either long-term or acute one-time exposure. This fact is of potential significance because many experts believe that certain enzyme deficiencies contribute to migraine, particularly dietary migraine, from which I suffer. Thus, I can build a circumstantial case for a chlordane–migraine link, a link not sufficient to cause me to vacate my residence, but enough to engage my interest and put me on the lookout for further information.

Of course, chlordane was the treatment of choice for termite control for many years, and for most of that time spraying the substance was a perfectly legal and acceptable method of application. Chlordane undoubtedly was sprayed under, around, and, regrettably, even inside many hundreds of thousands of homes, work places, and public buildings in this country. During that same time period, public policy encouraged us to tighten up our buildings' interiors as an energy-saving measure, thus assuring heightened exposure to this highly toxic chemical that vaporizes rapidly when heated.

I am extremely interested in hearing from any of you migraine sufferers who noticed either the beginning or worsening of your symptoms after some type of chlordane exposure. If you have noted such a possible connection, please write to me at the address given in Appendix D. If you like, include further details along with your name and address. I will answer all correspondence and, if the response justifies, will attempt to consolidate and appropriately follow up on the findings.

Legal Ramifications of Disabling Illness

Knowing whether you might qualify for such a dual diagnosis (multiple chemical sensitivity as well as migraine) could be important because both MCS and migraine may well be considered legal disabilities under the Americans with Disabilities Act (ADA), which was signed into law in July, 1991, with most key provisions becoming effective in July, 1992. Among other things, this law is intended to prohibit job discrimination against persons with disabilities. Currently, this protection applies only to firms with at least 25 employees; in July, 1994, it will cover those where 15 or more work. In addition, those employees falling under the scope of the law may, under specific circumstances, be entitled to special considerations in the work place, to certain housing modifications in the rental market, and, in cases of extreme disability, to Social Security benefits as well.

Either diagnosis, for instance, might well give a person valuable leverage with a landlord in forestalling potentially harmful property modifications, such as pesticide treatment or the installation of a new carpet. (Actually, both the Department of Housing and Urban Development [HUD] and the

Social Security Administration have already granted administrative recognition to MCS sufferers.)

Experts in the field of health law are only beginning to explore the impact that this new law will have on severe headache sufferers. It is already apparent, however, that the subjective nature of headache disorders can present obstacles when one pursues legal rights under the ADA. Working with knowledgeable doctors and attorneys would be essential in any such attempt, whether the disability be one of severe headache or MCS or both, because both conditions share a similar hard-to-define quality; and with both, proving exactly what factors cause symptoms is apt to be difficult.

In his 1991 book, *The Employee Rights Handbook,* experienced labor attorney Steven Mitchell Sack provides useful strategies for dealing with illegal health-related questions and requirements in job interviews. Sack also explains how to press for a smoke-free work environment.

The Big Picture: *Lifestyle Factors*

Admittedly this chapter has covered some very diverse territory. The unifying theme among the various topics discussed is the fact that all represent areas of individual lifestyle control for migraineurs. By appropriately addressing each of these areas, we can make significant strides toward reclaiming control of our lives. Keep reading for a discussion of other areas where corrective action will pay off.

Meanwhile consider the following lifestyle choices to maximize your odds against migraine:

1. Maintain a regular schedule of eating and sleeping.
2. Reduce internal stress by learning to identify and modify major stressors stemming from your personality, your past, your job, and your relationships.
3. Stimulate natural pain-relieving substances by learning relaxations skills and by participating in a regular aerobic exercise program.
4. Quit smoking and other tobacco use and minimize exposure to second-hand smoke.
5. Minimize or avoid exposure to toxic environmental chemicals.

Balance to Be Achieved

To minimize/eliminate migraine symptoms while still retaining a satisfying level of spontaneity in your life.

Chapter 5

The Impact of Diet

A Commonsense Approach

The Food–Headache Link: *Darkness Abounds*

If you changed the type of gasoline or oil you were putting in your car, and within the next few days the engine suddenly became loud and sluggish, what would be the first thing that crossed your mind? Pretty obvious, isn't it? Yet why do so few people give even a passing thought to their diets when they become ill or just feel less than their best? Well, guess what? Most of us migraineurs are no different from the next person when it comes to missing the rather obvious connection between diet and well-being. We all tend to take food pretty much for granted, and what we aren't on the lookout for, we just may fail to notice.

I think of my neighbor's daughter, who at the age of seven began to suffer from debilitating migraine attacks. When I asked her mom whether she had considered possible dietary triggers, the woman dismissed the very idea outright and with some indignation, almost as if I were challenging her maternal credentials. I gave her a migraine diet anyway. The next time we talked, she insisted that her daughter never ate chocolate or peanut butter. Quite an unusual kid, I thought to myself. A few months later, when the two of us happened to meet at a neighborhood gathering, the mom approached me rather sheepishly and admitted having discovered that her daughter had been drinking chocolate milk—both during her school lunches and at some Girl Scout meetings as well. When the child overindulged, a migraine attack invariably followed.

The low level of awareness among migraineurs about the role dietary triggers play in their disorder was demonstrated in 1975 by the British researcher, Dr. Katharina Dalton. Dalton surveyed the food and alcohol intake of more than 1800 female sufferers during the 24-hour period prior to naturally occurring migraine attacks. A significant number of the subjects had eaten either chocolate, cheese, citrus, and/or alcohol during that time, and a majority of the sufferers had missed meals. The author concluded that in only 5% of the subjects was there no dietary factor present, but only 16% of the sufferers themselves attributed their attacks to either food, alcohol, or fasting. Most blamed stress.

Doctors, too, are guilty of either ignoring, minimizing, or denying the migraine–food link; I have personally encountered all three of these attitudes. Two of my doctors casually presented me with a written migraine diet—one on her own initiative, the other only after I asked for it. Both of these diets consisted only of short lists of foods to avoid and were totally lacking in accompanying rationale, let alone suggestions for successful adherence. Additionally, although there was some overlap between the two, there were some striking inconsistencies as well. Two other doctors were far less helpful: One neurologist vociferously denied any dietary connection, and another responded to my request for dietary help with the advice that I would have to visit a headache clinic to receive such lifestyle guidance.

Of the numerous popular books and articles written on migraine in the past few years, none fully explores this dietary link; some dismiss it entirely. There is some justification for the confusion and lack of interest in this area of headache treatment on the part of medical personnel. Research is inconclusive, and physicians seldom are willing to set out on unproven waters these days. Careful evaluation of the major research findings, however, supports the position that a significant number of sufferers will benefit from specific dietary changes.

In a classic 1982 study, reviewer R. J. Kohlenberg concluded that many of the research studies investigating the diet–migraine link have been poorly designed and carried out; he goes on to emphasize that this important matter deserves a more systematic and intelligent approach. Unfortunately, the careful research that Kohlenberg calls for would be both difficult and costly, and the financial profits from doing it probably would not be great. For those reasons, dietary migraine remains a most neglected area.

Dietary Sensitivity: *Practitioners and Sufferers Speak*

Surveys of physicians specializing in headache treatment as well as the self-reports of migraine sufferers themselves estimate that 25–40% of migraineurs belong to a dietary subgroup—in other words, that as many as 25–40% of all sufferers, at least on occasion, experience attacks as a direct result of the foods they eat. Foods most often identified as troublemakers are the "three C's:" chocolate, cheese, and citrus.

Generally it is believed that foods play a more important role in triggering migraine in children than in adults. Of course, children often eat relatively large amounts of the foods that are most likely to bother migraineurs anyway—such things as hot dogs, peanut butter, pizza, and chocolate. Whether adult or child, food-sensitive individuals often can bring about dramatic reduction both in the frequency and severity of their symptoms by first identifying and then either restricting or avoiding the offending foods.

How can you tell whether you are such an individual—whether certain foods trigger some or all of your headaches? Perhaps you already have this personal awareness because you have observed an obvious cause–effect relationship between specific foods and the occurrence of attacks. Occasional bingeing on certain foods such as chocolate or alcohol, for example, or the special indulgence in a seasonal food like strawberries or fruitcake might send you a message that would be hard to miss. I will begin to help you detect any possible dietary triggers by relating the way I became aware of mine.

When my daughter and I started to experience painful migraine episodes, we had just added a new food to our diets—tofu, the cheese-like soybean curd so widely used in Oriental cuisine and now becoming popular elsewhere because it is both nutritious and low calorie. Spotting the connection between our tofu consumption and the onset of severe symptoms was a fairly simple matter.

In my case, another link became apparent around Christmas every year; with impressive regularity, I began to experience annually—coinciding with a seasonal visit from my in-laws—what at that time were my only really severe attacks. No, the reaction was not stress-related, for we had always had a very loving and pleasant relationship. However, my father-in-law was a coffee lover; and when he came, I indulged myself by joining with him in several cups of very strong coffee each day. In addition, I used their visit as an excuse to serve ham, a food that I ordinarily avoided because of its high sodium and fat content.

Several disastrous holiday seasons passed before I began to understand the real cause of my misery. Initially my doctors blamed stress, while I suspected an allergy to the Christmas tree! A food diary was the tool that finally allowed me to zero in on coffee and ham as the major culprits.

Spurred on by these initial insights into dietary triggers, I began to look into the possibility of a more comprehensive relationship between food and migraines. The picture that emerged from my research was far from clear; on the contrary, the headache–diet connection is both cloudy and complicated. I'm glad that I kept digging, however, for the search eventually paid off handsomely.

The Nature of the Dietary Connection: *What It Is and Isn't*

Experts neither pretend to fully understand nor are they unanimous in their current explanations about how certain foods act in the body to trigger a migraine attack. In general, relatively little is known about the extremely intricate biochemical processes that occur between the time a food is eaten and the time it is assimilated and/or eliminated by the body.

The biggest dietary troublemaker for migraineurs appears to be a family of nitrogen-based protein components called amines. Thus far researchers have identified at least seven of these potent amine family members that appear in our daily diets. These are:

- Dopamine, found in legumes, such as:
  - Peanuts
  - Peas
  - Broad beans and soy
- Tyramine, which forms as foods age, prevalent in products such as:
  - Cheese
  - Yogurt
  - Buttermilk
  - Sourdough
  - Wine
  - Dried or pickled meat and fish
- Histamine, appearing in cold-water fish, such as salmon and tuna
- Phenylethylamine, found in chocolate
- Octopamine and synephrine, occurring in citrus
- Tryptamine, present in tomatoes and pineapple.

As if these amine enemies don't give us enough trouble, our foods contain a whole host of other headache provokers. In general, any substance with vasoactive properties—that is, any ingredient that acts to constrict or dilate blood vessels—poses a threat to the well-being of food-sensitive migraineurs. In subsequent discussions of these agents, for the sake of brevity, they will be called simply "VAS" (short for vasoactive substances).

Other than the amines mentioned above, the chief offenders are caffeine and alcohol, as well as several ingredients added to our food by manufacturers. Included in the latter group are monosodium glutamate (MSG), the so-called flavor enhancer; aspartame, the artificial sweetener, usually sold as Nutrasweet (Equal); and for at least some of us, sulfite, a preservative that prevents discoloration. Preliminary evidence also implicates as possible VAS chemicals called phenols, which occur naturally in tea, coffee, and certain fruits and vegetables, as well as in most artificial food colorings.

As was mentioned earlier, there is some controversy about just how these VAS act in the body to produce a migraine attack. Some experts believe that diet-sensitive sufferers are deficient in one or more enzymes whose job it is to process VAS and render them harmless, as indeed they are in normal individuals. Investigations into such possible enzyme deficiencies have yielded mixed results. Complicating the job for researchers, the suspect trio of enzymes functions primarily in the liver and gastrointestinal tract, where levels are difficult to measure. Thus far, evaluations of their levels have been made primarily through blood measurements, which some authorities doubt to be a valid reflection of activity in other organs.

Other experts reject the enzyme-deficiency theory, instead attributing food sensitivities to other causes, chiefly to a general vascular instability and subsequent vulnerability to agents affecting that system. Whatever the exact mechanism, most agree that the food sensitivity leading to migraine attacks is *not* a food allergy.

Although some people use the term "allergy" when speaking of any sensitivity, this term, in its most technical, medical sense, is a very narrow one—referring only to a specific type of immune system reaction that involves mast cells. Headache authorities are nearly unanimous in the opinion that migraine reactions do not directly involve that system.

Be sure you and your doctor or dietitian are talking the same language on this important matter, or confusion can result. Tests, such as the RAST blood test or the scratch or interdermal tests, sometimes used to identify specific food allergens, are of absolutely no help in identifying this more general dietary sensitivity of migraineurs. Remember, too, that in investigating and identifying true allergens, one checks for problems with one food at a time.

In the case of migraine sensitivities, it is the total VAS load that counts; just as other headache triggers are cumulative in nature (as Chapter 3 emphasizes), so too are food triggers. One beer may not set off an attack in a particular person, whereas two or three may cause excruciating misery; likewise, one hot dog may do no harm to a given sufferer, unless it happens to be eaten with baked beans and onions and washed down with lemonade. The more VAS eaten, the more severe the reaction will be. The more sensitive the particular sufferer is to these substances, then the smaller the amount required to produce troublesome symptoms.

Allergies As Indirect Triggers: The Plot Thickens

The following information may, at first glance, seem to contradict the points just made about the difference between migraine sensitivities and allergic reactions. Please be patient; this matter is somewhat complex, but it is understandable.

Although the general dietary-migraine sensitivity is not an allergy, some migraineurs can have both actual food allergies and this general VAS sensitivity. When food allergies are present, then they in turn can trigger migraine attacks in those individuals. This is a controversial matter: Most, but certainly not all, experts hold this theory of the indirect allergy trigger.

Allow me to attempt to clarify this significant and often misunderstood relationship between allergies and migraine: Most migraineurs with dietary sensitivities do not have allergies—that is, do not have immune system mast cell reactions; adverse reactions in this majority of diet-sensitive sufferers are caused instead by an instability of the vascular system, possibly accompanied by an enzyme deficiency.

However, there are some sufferers, who in addition to this VAS sensitivity, also experience actual mast cell reactions. In this smaller group, some other symptom besides migraine usually occurs to signal the presence of the allergy. This could be hives, a rash, or swelling somewhere in the body, especially the throat or respiratory system. It is also important to realize that a true allergic reaction usually occurs relatively quickly after exposure, whereas the VAS response may be delayed for as long as 24 or even 36 hours.

The allergic reaction, in turn, can indirectly provoke a migraine attack, many experts believe, although admittedly they do not understand exactly how this secondary triggering action happens. The mechanism may be somewhat akin to the way a viral or bacterial infection sometimes triggers an attack. In a susceptible person, almost any significant biochemical upset seems to be a potential trigger. It may be helpful in understanding this indirect triggering event to compare the migraineur to the diabetic, another patient in whom almost any significant biochemical happening often worsens symptoms of the primary disease.

For people with both types of reactions—the immune system allergic response coupled with the more common VAS sensitivity—the trigger-identification process obviously will be more complicated. Not only will this class of migraineurs have to find their tolerable VAS loads, they will also need to identify individual food allergens. Unfortunately, even for this group, medical testing often proves of no help. Food-allergy tests are notoriously unreliable, or so my doctors tell me. Again the most valuable tool will be the food diary and, in this case, possibly a medically supervised elimination diet.

Reaction Variability: Sometimes Yes, Sometimes No

One of the most puzzling aspects of dietary management, according to many migraineurs, is the unpredictable reaction they experience to certain foods. Sometimes a sufferer will develop symptoms from eating onion, for example, but at other times will escape unscathed. Several factors come into play to help explain this rather peculiar state of affairs. The most obvious ones, of course, are serving size, and accompanying VAS—the total load. No doubt you've caught on to this by now.

Beyond the obvious, however, there are other considerations. In dealing with both tyramine, the protein component that forms during the aging process, and with mold, a very common allergen, variability can be expected, although certainly not predicted with any degree of exactness. If we eat foods prone to tyramine and mold buildup (*see* Level II chart later in this chapter), then, we really have to expect the unexpected. Applying the tests for food freshness suggested in a later note should help to minimize tyramine/mold ingestion, but unfortunately there is no foolproof way to avoid these substances completely—short of stopping eating, and that route certainly is not recommended.

Researchers report some interesting findings about the variability of tyramine formation in food. In two pieces of aged cheese that look and taste exactly the same, for example, tyramine content may vary as much as 100-fold, making reaction predictability an exceptionally poor gamble. The tyramine content of alcoholic beverages likewise varies tremendously, with great differences even among various batches of the same varieties of beer and wine produced by the same manufacturer.

When puzzling over reaction variability, don't neglect the role of internal setting, or threshold, which was discussed in Chapter 3 in regard to general triggers. In female sufferers, the most common causes of trigger vulnerability are cyclical estrogen dips. This matter is discussed in detail in Chapter 7; let's just say here that many women seem to be most sensitive to triggers during times when estrogen levels are falling. Because many of us experience exaggerated dietary reactions just prior to or during our menstrual periods, we can often benefit greatly from a stricter dietary program at that time. In addition, some sufferers may note increased dietary sensitivity during times of long-term stress, letdown, or unusual fatigue, and may profit from greater dietary vigilance during those times.

When evaluating food reactions, remember to allow for the lag time—as much as 24–36 hours, but more commonly between three and 14—that can elapse between the time a food is eaten and the time symptoms appear. This is a matter that confounds dietary detection work for many migraineurs and one of the main reasons for keeping a written record of food eaten. Patterns tend to become much more obvious when recorded in black and white.

Some experts believe that many, if not all, sufferers experience a short period of immunity immediately following an attack—a period of two or three days during which, no matter what the trigger exposure, no further attacks will occur. That factor, too, may possibly explain some instances of reaction variability. (My personal experience does not confirm such an immunity, but perhaps others' may. I have found that continued trigger exposure results in a worsening of symptoms even if I have just recovered from an attack.)

To summarize, then, the following factors should be considered in attempting to understand unpredictability of food reactions:

1. Total VAS load consumed
2. Varied amine, mold, or additive content of food
3. Differing internal setting, e.g., hormone fluctuations, fatigue, or the presence of other triggers
4. Period of possible immunity immediately following an attack

Seeking A Personal Safety Zone: Sherlock Holmes at Work

Unfortunately there are no easy or even guaranteed ways to tell whether some or all of your attacks are triggered by foods, beverages, or additives. Dietary migraine programs are similar to diabetes regimens in their overall design and goals; but unlike diabetics, we are not given handy little measuring devices or carefully devised plans for assuring safe food intake. To date no lab tests have been devised to accomplish this purpose; and, alas, as already implied, most doctors are quite unsophisticated about providing guidance in this area.

Your own trained observations and instincts are likely to be your biggest assets in finding your personal safety zone. Persistent effort is required in this detective work. Before you make any dietary changes, however, it still is important to seek professional guidance to be sure that your general nutritional requirements are met and that other medical conditions are not worsened.

The VAS Total Load Approach

The rest of this chapter and the following one focus on helping you not only to locate your personal dietary safety zone, but also to live within it as easily and happily as possible. I call this approach to dietary migraine management "The VAS Total Load Approach." Although I coined that particular phrase, the theory behind it is grounded solidly in the research and opinions of migraine experts, including British researchers Drs. Edda Hanington and Maurice Lessof, and the educational materials circulated by ACHE, a major US headache support organization, among others.

The particular load that creates problems depends entirely on the degree of sensitivity of the individual sufferer. Since few of us want to give up any more foods than we absolutely must in order to control our symptoms, the trick here is to identify the load that we as individuals can tolerate. The various VAS levels presented in chart form later in this chapter will provide a place to start in that process, but such personal identification definitely will require both trial and error as well as careful planning on your part. Keeping a food diary probably will be your most important aid.

The Diary: A Key to Success

In order to use this or any other dietary management program, you will need a food diary or journal; a simple notebook will do very nicely. Decide where you most conveniently can make regular entries—kitchen table, bedside stand, or lounge chair, for example—and then firmly plant your notebook there with a pen attached. You have at least two options for making food entries, and you will need to decide which method better suits your lifestyle and temperament. If you have a regular schedule and tend to approach things systematically, perhaps you will be willing to make daily journal entries, either after each meal (probably the safest way) or at least at the end of each day.

If that method sounds too boring or burdensome, you may take a short cut. One effective method for someone having headaches no more than once a week is to make an entry at the first sign of a headache, recording all foods and beverages (including both meals and snacks) consumed during the prior 36-hour period. In order to assure best results, you should do this before your pain becomes severe; otherwise you may omit something important. This second option is called backtracking.

Whichever you choose, the daily entry or backtracking method, consistency and willingness to spend time evaluating entries to identify food–symptom connections will be essential for success. This means that you will need to record not only foods eaten, but also headaches or other migraine symptoms experienced, and attempt to recognize any possible connection between the two. If you are hesitant to try this evaluation process on your own, or you get stuck somewhere along the way, ask your mate, a fellow migraineur, or your dietitian for assistance. Sometimes an extra set of eyes can be quite helpful.

If you are just beginning your diary, review Chapter 3 so that you can include information about other possible triggers and threshold setters along with your food entries for a comprehensive picture of your migraine situation. For still more tips about possible culprits, read Chapters 6 through 9 before you actually begin making entries. The suggested format in Appendix A allows for a comprehensive but simple approach to diary-keeping.

The Individual and Dietary Management

There are many reasonable ways to use this dietary-management program. Your individual situation and lifestyle will determine whether you use the program at all, and if so, how.

Just how closely you adhere to any migraine management regimen will be determined, at least in part, by how much of a risk-taker you are. For example, a generally cautious person will not chance suffering an attack, especially if symptoms are severe, whereas a gambler may venture forth into unknown dietary territory whenever the whim strikes, with fingers crossed that unpleasant consequences will be escaped—at least until the wager is lost. Obviously only the individual involved can decide whether or not an indiscretion is worth the risk.

Allow me to outline some factors to keep in mind when selecting a beginning level and some ways I foresee each level as being used. These suggestions are based on my personal experience, the experiences of acquaintances, and in-depth research—all tempered with some common sense!

Level I

A person who currently experiences annoying but not debilitating attacks might wish to begin simply by avoiding the worst offending foods. Concurrently this individual might choose to keep a 24-hour backtracking type of food diary to gain insight into any other food triggers, and to note any dietary transgressions and resulting symptoms. This might be someone who is on preventive medication, someone who has found a personally effective migraine-aborting medication that she feels comfortable using, or simply someone whose symptoms are not severe.

The foods listed in the Level I chart are widely recognized as the most troublesome for diet-sensitive migraineurs. Some sufferers can banish most, or even all, of their attacks by avoiding these items—not so easy as it may first appear, primarily because of the wide use of MSG in our processed foods.

Level II

This level of dietary control might well be a reasonable starting point for many of you who are trying to determine possible food sensitivity. For you, a trial period of about six weeks should be enlightening—coupled, of course, with the diary-keeping method of your choice. Unless such a trial is well planned and conscientiously followed, however, it—like some of the research studies—will neither prove nor disprove anything.

A person who wishes to avoid all medication, either because of pregnancy or for other medical reasons, or one who has found no effective, tolerable migraine-preventive or -abortive medication may choose to adhere to

Level 1
Worst Offenders

Food	Comments/examples
Aged cheese	All except American, Farmer's, creamed, and cottage
Alcohol	Especially red wine
Caffeine	In excessive amounts (more than two 5-oz. cups of coffee or tea per day)
Chocolate	All forms, including chocolate milk
Citrus	Grapefruit, lemons, limes, and oranges
Cured meats	Bacon, ham, all types of sausage, including pepperoni and hot dogs; and deli meats
Legumes	Broad beans, such as kidney, navy, and others; lentils; peas; peanuts; and soy
Monosodium glutamate (MSG)	Bouillion, most commercial soups and gravies, prepared entrees, and canned tuna (*see* Chapter 6 for other common sources.)
Aspartame (Nutrasweet™/ Equal™)	In many artificially sweetened commercial products, such as soft drinks, desserts, and so forth

the most stringent version of this level on a semipermanent basis. In conjunction with the required restrictions, an all-out effort might be made, at least for the first two months, by keeping a daily food diary and recording entries after each meal.

Another type of migraineur for whom this level might well be appropriate is the female who notices that most of her headaches, or at least her most severe ones, occur at a particular phase of her menstrual cycle; such a woman would likely benefit from strict adherence to this level if only during that time of heightened susceptibility. Normal eating patterns could be resumed during the remainder of the month, if she so chooses.

This level also might represent a reasonable starting place for a sufferer experiencing moderate to severe symptoms who fails to gain satisfactory relief from other measures. A person using this level of control may or may not choose also to eliminate the most common remaining allergens: wheat, eggs, milk, corn, and oats.

The listing of foods in the Level II chart not only suggests what foods to avoid when adhering to Level II, but also explains the reasons for that avoidance.

As you can plainly see, this list is formidable. As a person who loves to eat—in fact one who lives to eat rather than eating to live, as perhaps it should be—I am not suggesting for one minute that you completely swear

Level II
Potent Headache Provokers

Food group	Items restricted
Beverages	Alcohol (M;P;S;Ty); chocolate milk and cocoa (Ph); coffee, sodas (brown and others containing caffeine), and tea (C;P); Ovaltine and Postum (malt); ginseng
Cereals	All bran, added bran (any grain); malt-flavored
Dairy products	Buttermilk, cheese (all except American and cottage), sour cream, and yogurt (Na-Ty)
Fruits and juices	Citrus (NA-O); dried (all, including coconut) (M;S;Ty); grapes (M;P;S); Maraschino cherries (S); melon (NA-UNK); papayas (NA-UNK); pineapple (N-T); plums (NA-UNK); raspberries (M;NA-UNK); and strawberries (M;NA-UNK)
Protein	Cured meats (bacon, Canadian bacon, cold cuts and most deli meats, corned beef, ham, pressed turkey and turkey roasts, sausage, including pepperoni) (M;MSG;N;Ty); dried, smoked, or pickled meat and fish (including barbecue, caviar, and anchovies) (M;MSG;N;Ty); marinated meats (MSG, soy); organ meats (including all kinds of liver) (NA-Ty); cold-water fish (H); and prebasted poultry (MSG;S); peanuts and peanut butter (D); soy protein (including hydrolyzed vegetable protein or HVP) (D;MSG)
Vegetables	Avocados and guacamole (NA-UNK); broad beans (including pole, Italian broad, garbanzo, navy, white, lima, butter and kidney) (D); eggplant (especially the peel); garlic (Ty); lentils (D); mushrooms (M;Ty); onions (M;Ty); peas (black-eyed, green English, snow, and sugar snap) (D); potato products containing sulfites (some canned, dried, and frozen); red cabbage; sauerkraut (M;Ty); tomatoes (NA-T)
Condiments	Commercial salad dressings, barbecue sauce, catsup, and mustard (except in very small quantities) (MSG;Ty); pickles and olives (S;Ty); sauces (soy, teriyaki, worcestershire, or steak) (D;Ty); vinegar (all except white distilled) (Ty)

(continued)

Abbreviations: C, caffeine; D, dopamine; H, histamine; NA, natural amines; MSG, monosodium glutamate; M, mold; N, nitrites; O, octopamine; P, phenols; Py, phehyl-alanine; S, sulfites; Ty, tyramine; Rd/Ty, rapidly deteriorating/tyramine; T, tryptamine; UNK, unknown.

Level II *(continued)*

Food group	Items restricted
Miscellaneous	Aspartame (Nutrasweet™/Equal™); chocolate; carob; (a chocolate substitute) (D); commercial ice-cream, pudding, and cottage cheese thickened with vegetable gums (D); natural licorice (D); malt, papaya-based meat tenderizers (NA-UNK); seaweed/carrageenan (D;MSG); sourdough bread (M;Ty); soy flour (D); yeast extracts (like Marmite) (M;Ty); any commercially prepared foods with unknown ingredients (MSG;S;Ty)

off all of these foods. But, if you want to minimize pain, you need to look carefully at your consumption of any and all of them. Remember, it's the total VAS load that counts!

We all wish there were some magic formula for accurately gaging just exactly how many of these offenders we might safely consume, but, alas, there is no such animal. A conscientiously kept food diary is the best available tool for making such an assessment. If, however, you are experiencing debilitating symptoms, or simply cannot bear the possibility of another attack, then the only completely safe strategy really is total avoidance of these troublemakers.

Level III

This extremely restrictive program (*see* Level III chart) is appropriate only as a temporary measure, under medical supervision. It constitutes what the allergists call an elimination diet and is meant to be a last resort by which desperate sufferers, who cannot bear the thought of one more attack, can begin to get a handle on their food triggers. This level can likewise help those daily headache sufferers who suspect they have multiple food sensitivities/allergies that they are unable to identify on less restrictive diets. (Migraineurs first should be sure that they are not abusing medications known to cause rebound headache, including simple pain relievers, such as aspirin and Tylenol; ergot derivatives; barbiturates like butalbital; and caffeine. *See* Chapter 9 for more information about this topic.)

In order to make this program work, a very conscientious meal-by-meal diary should accompany it. The idea here is to adhere strictly to the diet for at least one full week and then to begin adding other foods, at a rate of no more than two per week, while continuing to avoid all foods listed in Level II.

This elimination diet is neither as simple to use nor as effective in identifying VAS triggers as it is in identifying true food allergies, the purpose for which it originally was designed. The strategy may be particularly helpful in

Level III
Generally Safe Foods

Food group	Items allowed
Beverages	Water only
Cereals/grains	Rice only
Condiments	Salt, distilled white vinegar, and vegetable oil
Fruits	Apples, peaches, and pears (peeled)
Protein	Very fresh beef, lamb, and chicken*
Vegetables	Beets, bell peppers, carrots, celery, cucumber, iceberg lettuce (discard outer leaves), potatoes (peeled), radishes, rutabagas, squash (all varieties), and turnips

*If you have a known allergy to milk, then the safest course would be to avoid beef during this trial period; likewise, if you are allergic to eggs, it would be best to avoid chicken.

identifying unknown food allergies that indirectly contribute to the migraine process, however. If you have reason to believe that you are experiencing actual food allergies (usually symptoms other than migraine will be present), then you may want to talk to your doctor about starting with some version of this level.

These foods contain few, if any, vasoactive ingredients. They are also uncommon allergens; however, it is possible for a given individual to be allergic to any food. The strictest elimination diet consists only of lamb, rice, distilled water, and a nonallergenic vitamin/mineral supplement; but such a diet would be so boring that probably only the most desperate sufferers would consider it.

Migraine and Vegetarianism: *An Uneasy Alliance*

Vegetarian migraineurs with dietary triggers will have a difficult time working out a sound nutritional plan—especially in light of the need for a high protein intake to forestall low blood sugar. In fact, for the strict vegan (one who eats no fish, eggs, or dairy products), developing such a plan is likely to be so difficult that a registered dietitian should be consulted. Vegetarians with food allergies or other medical conditions that further limit food choices, or who just plain dislike a large number of foods, will probably need professional help as well. A less strict vegetarian who does not suffer complicating considerations probably can meet personal protein requirements with milk, cottage and American cheese, eggs, some nuts and seeds, whole grain cereals (including wheat germ), breads, and pasta, and hearty vegetables such as acorn squash, white potatoes, sweet potatoes, and corn. The total ban on legumes (including all broad beans, peas, soy, and peanut products) required of most dietary migraineurs represents the greatest loss for the vegetarian, because these foods offer the most nearly complete vegetable protein as well as an impressive versatility of preparation.

Now that you have some tools for exploring possible dietary triggers, you are ready to go on to the next chapter, which provides specific practical tips for making a migraine diet work.

The Big Picture: *Diet as a Factor in Migraine*

1. Only your doctor and/or a registered dietitian can provide complete and definitive information about personal nutritional requirements.
2. A significant number of sufferers have dietary triggers, but these often go unrecognized.
3. Food sensitivities involved in migraine are not the same as food allergies, although sometimes allergic reactions also can trigger migraine attacks.
4. A family of dietary chemicals called amines, contained in many common foods, constitutes one set of primary triggers; preservatives and artificial sweeteners represent other frequent troublemakers.
5. Dietary factors in migraine tend to be complex and rather unpredictable.
6. A lag time from three to 36 hours may occur between eating a vasoactive substance and your reaction to it.
7. Total VAS is a key concept; foods act in combination, and the total amount consumed is more critical than any particular food(s).
8. A food diary is the best tool for identifying dietary triggers.
9. Each dietary-sensitive individual will have a slightly different personal safety zone—a different VAS load required to trigger symptoms—and this will vary with time and other trigger exposure.
10. In women, hormone levels are a primary determinant of dietary sensitivity, with the most vulnerable time usually occurring shortly before and/or during menstrual periods.

Chapter 6

Your Migraine Diet

Understanding and Hanging On

Examining Migraine Diets and Challenging the Experts

In examining well over a dozen migraine diets, I had two major concerns: (1) significant inconsistencies regarding which foods should be minimized or avoided, and (2) a lack of explicit rationale and guidelines.

Figuring out the rationale behind many of the available diets is a job for a rocket scientist or some equally bright professional, since often very little, if any, explanatory material is included. This lack of explanation and guidelines for successful adherence makes dietary management an extremely daunting, if not impossible, task for even the most motivated migraineur, and impatient or less motivated sufferers are apt to throw up their hands in total frustration after reading a couple of these "aids."

For example, one of the more helpful versions disallows cream and ice cream, but lists whipped cream as acceptable. Maybe there's a good reason for such a distinction; but no explanation is offered, and it's far from obvious. (Perhaps if very cold foods trigger your headaches, then this rationale might make sense; but we really shouldn't have to guess, should we?) The same diet permits whole wheat bread but disallows white bread; now granted, whole wheat is the more nutritious product by far, but the direct relevance of such a distinction remains a mystery. I could go on, but I won't; I think you see my point. Probably most of us can follow a diet more successfully and happily if we understand where it's coming from.

Inconsistencies/Deficiencies

The diets surveyed were either confusing or totally silent about the following important matters:

Bananas

Most diets disallow; I eat in moderation, being careful not to select over-ripe fruit. It's my understanding that most of the amines are in the peel, and even Chuckie, the chimp, passes those up. One small one daily is probably quite safe for most sufferers.

Bran

Never mentioned in migraine diets, this food is potentially risky because, as the outer layer of whatever grain, it is most likely to contain both mold and tyramine. Therefore, many sufferers will find they must avoid either all-bran cereals or cereals that contain added bran, or both. This includes such things as oat bran, 40% bran flakes, and all of the popular high fiber cereals that are so good for us in so many other ways. I eat whole grain cereals, such as shredded and puffed wheat, but avoid all with added bran. This is one I really had to learn the hard way. I kept trying to return to these so-called "healthy" cereals, but I got symptoms every single time. (Theoretically one could get into trouble eating even the whole grains [without added bran], but I suspect it's unlikely unless such grains make up a large part of the diet.) I limit my daily servings of whole grain products to three; wheat germ is a freebie—not counted in this total.

Citrus

Some diets forbid citrus entirely, while others allow in moderate amounts, e.g., 1/2 cup of orange juice daily. I have found citrus to be a potent trigger; and although it is important nutritionally, I consider it unsafe and take low-dose Vitamin C supplements instead.

Dairy Products

Some diets allow no cheese except cottage, whereas others permit American, cream, and/or farmer's. For years I ate only cottage. The tyramine content of any aged cheese tends to be quite unpredictable. Some diets allow 1/2 cup servings of yogurt; I continue to have unpleasant symptoms every time I try this, either in regular or frozen form (and I do love it so). Most frozen yogurt contains vegetable gums, also apt to cause migraine symptoms.

Milk is forbidden by a few diets; unless an allergy or lactose intolerance (inability to digest milk sugar) is present, there is no good reason for avoiding this nutritious dairy product. (Specific symptoms besides the typical migraine ones should clue a person into the presence of these other conditions; bloating, excess gas, and diarrhea, for example, usually signal the lactose intolerance, whereas a true allergy would be accompanied by such things as a rash or hives.)

Exotic Fruits

New fruits are being introduced into American supermarkets nearly every week, it seems. Few are addressed in traditional migraine diets. Kiwi, now one of the more familiar, is disallowed by some diets, and I avoid it. I recently made the happy discovery that I can enjoy rhubarb without problem. (Cherries, on the other hand—hardly exotic, I know—bother me.)

Fruit Juice

Apple and cranberry are probably the safest bets; all juices carry some risk, however, because damaged fruit is often included, bringing possible tyramine and mold contamination.

Grapes

Not usually mentioned; risky because of phenolic compounds in skin and frequent sulfite treatment. If eaten at all, do so very sparingly, avoiding the overripe or those removed from stems. Peeling the fruit should help if you have the patience. The same cautions apply to grape juice, which may be even riskier because mushy fruit is probably thrown into the vat.

Melon

Most diets do not mention this fruit; some advise caution. Avoid if overripe or if the outer shell has been damaged. I do better with watermelon than with either cantaloupe or honeydew, both of which often give me symptoms.

Mushrooms

Not usually mentioned, but risky because of frequent mold and probable tyramine content. If eaten, the whiter and fresher, the better.

Nuts/Seeds

Disallowed by most diets; I eat up to one ounce a day of either almonds, pecans, or sunflower seeds. Watch out for added MSG. (Avoid peanuts, which are really a legume and not a nut at all, because of their high dopamine content.)

Pineapple/Tomatoes

Diets are inconsistent. Although possibly less dangerous than citrus, these are potentially troublesome, at least in large quantities. I eliminated these for years, but now eat them in small amounts for occasional garnish or flavoring.

Pork

Disallowed by some diets, but without a clear rationale. My hunch is that the reactions experienced when eating cured pork were attributed by sufferers to the meat itself. I eat it rarely—because of the high fat content of most cuts—without apparent ill effect. Frequent consumption likely would contribute to undesirable blood platelet stickiness in the long run. (*See* the note on dietary fats, page 95, for a more complete explanation.)

Turkey

Turkey is high in tryptophan, an amino acid that our bodies convert into serotonin. On theoretical grounds, then, this food should be good for migraineurs. Some even tout turkey as a natural migraine abortive, if it is eaten in large quantities very early in an attack. On the other hand, some migraine diets forbid the food. You might try a little experimentation here, but be sure you're eating a preservative-free bird of relatively fresh quality. I notice that when I go really heavy on the turkey (Thanksgiving leftover week, for example), I tend to have more of my "little" headaches.

Seafood

Some diets disallow seafood. Although no doubt there are several potential problems with this food category, certain varieties can be eaten safely under carefully controlled conditions. One of the greatest perils faced here is the freshness factor; in a recent Consumers Union survey of seafood in Chicago and New York (published in the February, 1992, issue of *Consumer Reports* magazine), 40% of all samples tested were either spoiled or nearly spoiled. And it's no wonder. When the samples were taken from specialty shops or supermarkets, an average of 15 days had elapsed since the seafood had been reeled in. Cooking will usually destroy most of the harmful bacteria, but it will *not* destroy the troublesome tyramine.

The riskiest fish are those that are high in the amino acid histidine. (Our bodies convert it to histamine.) Included in this category are cold-water varieties, such as salmon, tuna, and mackerel, that produce histidine as a kind of natural antifreeze. Among the safest varieties of finfish (if fresh or fresh-frozen), are catfish (especially farm-raised), flounder, grouper, and halibut.

In addition to these issues, remember to watch for MSG in canned seafood. As of this writing, most canned fish harbors the additive under the guise of hydrolyzed vegetable protein (HVP). If the label lists anything other than fish, water, and salt, then the contents are open to suspicion.

There is yet another consideration: Frozen shell and finfish are often treated with sulfites, or another troublesome preservative called sodium tripolyphosphate. *See* my notes under "Sulfites" in this section (page 82) and under "Restaurant Meals" in a later section (page 97). Many cafeterias and buffet-style restaurants serve frozen, preservative-laden fish, especially cod.

Spinach

A few diets eliminate spinach; others allow or ignore it. Problems are likely to stem (pardon the pun) from blemished and deteriorating leaves. If fresh, examine the underside of the leaves for signs of mold or deterioration. Canned or frozen forms, in which quality cannot be verified, are risky.

Sugar

Because sugar tends to destabilize blood sugar levels, causing them to rise rapidly and then fall, and such fluctuating levels are a possible headache trigger, sugar binges definitely should be avoided. It's unwise to eat sweets in place of a meal or even in between meals; save them instead for dessert, to be eaten in moderate servings after appropriate amounts of protein and fiber. This strategy takes care of the blood sugar stabilization problem for most of us, and completely sacrificing sugar, as one migraine author recommends, is not necessary. What a bleak prospect!

Yeast

This a confusing matter. Most diets allow commercially baked bread, but disallow homemade yeast products, at least freshly baked items. The concern seems to be about the tyramine in the yeast; and I suppose the assumption made is that this ingredient is destroyed by the baking/cooling process—an assumption that I cannot confirm. It has been my experience that tyramine is not destroyed by cooking in protein items, such as chicken that has begun to spoil, and I see no reason that yeast should be any different.

At any rate, there are relatively small amounts of yeast in baked goods. I eat them in moderation without worrying whether they are made commercially or at home. Yeast extracts, such as the Marmite seasoning popular in Britain, are very concentrated and should be avoided, as should sourdough products, which have higher quantities of fermented ingredients than regular yeast goods.

Food Colorings

Not mentioned in migraine diets, these additives nevertheless have been shown in research to be potent destroyers of one of the enzymes that may be in short supply in migraineurs. It would be rather risky to make artificially colored soft drinks, gelatin desserts, or any similar product a regular part of one's diet. This could be an especially important consideration in children, who tend to consume large amounts of canned and powdered beverages, candy, and gelatin. Sensitive individuals also may react to tartrazine, a yellowish orange powder, occurring naturally in aspirin, and used as a coloring in other drugs.

Malt

This flavoring is risky because it is aged in a way that encourages the development of both mold and tyramine. It is often used in such everyday products as cereals (including Nutrigrain, Grapenuts, and many others) and pretzels, as well as in drink mixes (like Ovaltine).

Sulfites

This family of chemical preservatives and color protectors has received a lot of bad press in recent years because of a serious, sometimes even fatal, reaction it causes in asthmatics. This same chemical can also cause problems for others, and in spite of the peril it poses, it is still around. I suffer violent migraine symptoms whenever I inadvertently ingest this chemical, but it's never mentioned in migraine diets. The headache literature, however, cites the substance as a common trigger. Quite a few canned and packaged foods contain some form of sulfite. Fortunately it appears on the label in some fairly recognizable fashion, such as sodium sulfite (or bisulfite), sulfur dioxide, or potassium bisulfite (or metabisulfite).

Federal regulation now bans the use of sulfites on salad bar fixings, but restaurants can continue to serve it to unknowing customers, chiefly in shellfish and dried and frozen potato products, such as fries and hash browns. Containers in which these items are delivered to restaurant kitchens are supposed to indicate the presence of the ingredient. We can certainly ask the chef or server whether the establishment is serving us sulfited foods, but I'm not confident we will always get an accurate answer. I became quite ill recently after eating lobster at one of our area's finest seafood restaurants, where I mistakenly assumed that I would not be served a sulfite-treated product. Now I inquire specifically before ordering, speaking directly to the manager or chef rather than relying on the server to relay this critical message.

The following foods often contain sulfites: shellfish; dried fish, such as cod; all dried fruits, including coconut and fruitcake combinations; wine, wine coolers, beer, wine vinegar, and cider; Maraschino cherries; fruit juices or pie fillings (canned); frozen, dried, or canned potatoes (including virtually all instant mashed); avocado dip and guacamole; sauerkraut; hominy grits; soups (canned or dried), sauces, and gravies; and pickles/relish. Fortunately sulfite is now banned on raw produce, with the exception of grapes, where it still can be used as a fungicide. (And I wonder about bing cherries, which often inexplicably seem to give me problems.)

Considering the chemical's high potential for causing dangerous reactions, you may find it puzzling to learn that many drugs contain sulfites as well. (For a discussion of this preservative in various medications, *see* Chapter 9.)

Vegetable Gums

These products—often used as stabilizers and thickening agents in ice cream, puddings, powdered drink mixes, soups, and salad dressings, as well as many other prepared products—are members of the legume family and therefore pose a serious threat to us migraineurs. Regrettably, low-fat or fat-free products (salad dressings and frozen desserts) tend to contain larger amounts of these thickeners. Be on the lookout for them under these designations: carrageenan (or seaweed), cellulose, or karaya; or guar, arabic, tragacanth, or xanthan gums. Traditionally ignored in migraine diets, these agents have been described and evaluated in allergy articles, where I learned about them quite by accident.

Knowledge of these gums has explained a number of my previously mysterious reactions to such products as commercial ice cream; as long as I restrict myself to natural products without gum additives, I have no problem. Gums also may be troublesome when inhaled while using certain grooming products, such as hair spray, mousse, and setting lotion. I have developed head rushes and other unpleasant symptoms when using some of these cosmetics, as well as from reading freshly printed newspapers whose ink contains vegetable gums. Some dental adhesives also contain these ingredients.

Benzoate

Few diets advise avoidance of the preservative benzoate, although the headache literature cites it as a common trigger. Many soft drinks contain benzoate, sometimes called sodium benzoate or benzoic acid, and these may well represent the most likely source of troublesome amounts in the average diet.

Personally Adverse Reactions: From Left Field?

During the years when my symptoms were most severe, I had trouble with some foods that are generally regarded as safe, or at least not mentioned in migraine diets. The following were my enemies:

Crucifers: Broccoli, Cauliflower, and Brussel Sprouts

I frequently seem to have problems with these otherwise very healthful foods. I doubt I was ever allergic to them because I could always eat kale, another member of this cabbage or crucifer family, with no problem at all. (Red cabbage is cited by some researchers as being high in phenols; I avoid it for that reason.) I might have been reacting to chemical pesticides sprayed on these other crucifers or to mold or tyramine that builds up in their moist

closed surfaces as they age—either on the grocery store shelves or somewhere between California and my dinner table. I do better with the frozen than the so-called fresh versions, although sometimes I react badly
even to the former.

Corn and Corn Products

If I eat more than one average serving within a 36 hour period, I get into
trouble with corn, corn bread, or popcorn. One source suggests that it blocks
the effects of serotonin because corn is high in the amino acid leucine.

Oat Products

I have a similar problem with oat products when eaten to excess. (I can't
find any definitive information linking oats to migraine, but interestingly,
my daughter has the same grain sensitivity.)

What I Ate: A Personal Adaptation

Working within the Level II framework, I developed the following personal dietary regimen, one fitting my lifestyle and personal preferences in
addition to accommodating my VAS Load limit. Now that I take both hormone supplements and a preventive medication, I have been able to relax
these restrictions somewhat, but in order to feel well I still must watch
what I eat quite closely. The following reflects the original, fairly strict
version of my dietary program, one that I followed during the years when
my attacks were most severe.

> *Beverages:* Postum, Seven-Up, diluted apple and cranberry juices, some
> weak herb teas in moderation (no ginseng), and decaf (one or two cups
> daily)
>
> *Cereals:* Cream of Wheat with wheat germ; shredded wheat; Breakfast
> Spiced Rice*; puffed wheat or rice with added wheat germ, sliced
> almonds, and/or bananas
>
> *Dairy products:* Sweet milk, 1/2 and 1% butterfat; low-fat cottage cheese
> (without vegetable gums); eggs (2 per week, limited only out of concern
> for fat content); margarine in moderation
>
> *Fruits:* Apples, apricots, bananas (one small per day), peaches, pears, and
> rhubarb; blueberries, cranberries, and melon in small amounts; fresh or
> frozen coconut
>
> *Grains/breads:* Barley (not malted), rice (brown and white); any bread
> without soy flour or sourdough; Triscuits; plain rice cakes; selected
> bagels, pancakes, and waffles (no soy flour or malt) wheat germ as
> desired. Whole grains limited to three servings daily; wheat germ need

not be included in total. (No cereals or breads with extra bran or malt added; no oatmeal.)

Protein foods: Any fresh lean poultry, beef, lamb, pork, or finfish (other than cold-water varieties); fresh frozen finfish; Gerber's Meat Sticks. Almonds, pecans, or sunflower seeds, 1 oz. daily total. (No shellfish except selected live lobster.)

Vegetables: Asparagus, beets, cabbage, carrots, corn (1/2 cup twice a week), kale (fresh only), okra (frozen only), potatoes, rutabagas, spinach (fresh only), squash (all varieties), string beans, sweet potatoes, turnips, water chestnuts, wax beans, lettuce (all varieties), bell peppers, celery, cucumbers, and radishes

Condiments: Distilled white vinegar and olive oil with herbs; very small amounts of mustard, ketchup, pickles/relish, horseradish, commercial salad dressings; barbecue sauce (Bull's-Eye original style only)

Desserts: Graham crackers, vanilla wafers, ginger snaps, sugar cookies; angel food cake; apple bread pudding*; pumpkin custard*; apple, peach, or pumpkin pie (occasionally); vanilla pudding (with added coconut or banana); natural ice-milk; pecan pie (rarely)

Snacks: Pretzels (no malt flavoring), plain potato chips (no MSG); popcorn in small amounts; Triscuits or any crackers without soy flour or MSG. (2 ounces of whole grain crackers counted as 1 serving.)

Can We Talk?

A great deal of information is presented in this chapter. It wouldn't be surprising if you are feeling somewhat overwhelmed just about now. Not to worry. Probably a rereading or two will be required—in addition to a little time to begin to mentally digest everything. Make some notes for yourself, if you think that might help, and don't neglect to use the food charts provided for your convenience in Appendix F.

Quite honestly, changing our eating patterns is seldom pleasant. You should know going into this program that developing and carrying out your own effective and nutritionally sound migraine management diet will require some mental effort, persistence, and probably some psychological discomfort as well. Most of us have many long-held food preferences; like other habits, these are not easy to break. Moreover, we use foods for psychological as well as physical reasons—not only to nourish our bodies, but also to comfort ourselves in times of fatigue, frustration, sadness, and anger. Those are just a few of the reasons we find changing our food habits diffi-

*Recipes included in Appendix E.

cult. In a migraine management program, however, the potential rewards are so great that I encourage you to regard this task as a challenge and get to work.

Specific Information About Dietary Migraine

The following topical comments gleaned from my experience, networking, and research are offered to assist you in your personal dietary management program. This is the type of crucial guidance that is either woefully lacking or entirely missing in most so-called migraine diets. I had to dig deeply to discover much of it, enduring much frustration in the process. I am eager to share it with you.

The Freshness Factor: Critical but Neglected

Although traditionally overlooked, food freshness is essential for migraineurs. In selecting foods our senses must be highly discriminatory. Such strictness is necessary because tyramine, considered by many authorities to be the most potent of the edible VAS, multiplies rapidly as foods age. The formation of this amino acid begins long before foods would be judged spoiled by conventional standards. For example, slightly deteriorating foods, such as overripe bananas, soft berries, or bruised spinach leaves, which would not harm the average person, could be enough to trigger an attack in a sensitive individual. A tough standard is definitely called for here.

Tyramine formation occurs most rapidly under the same conditions that encourage mold development—that is, after food has been crushed, bruised, or stored in damp places where little air circulates. My experience tells me that neither cooking nor freezing destroys tyramine that has already formed, although either process will halt further development of the amine. Here are some ways to assure food freshness:

Produce

1. Select slightly underripe items.
2. Pick fruits and vegetables with few, if any, cuts, bruises, or discolored spots. (Examine greens on the underside of the leaves.)
3. Avoid visible rust, mold, or slime.
4. Buy loose rather than prepackaged items if available, to allow closer inspection and avoid excessive moisture.
5. At home, open any prepackaged produce; before refrigerating, arrange for packaging that allows some ventilation; if excessively wet, wrap items in paper towels before repackaging.

6. Before eating, generously trim away any questionable areas. Avoid items that become soft or spongy, develop an alcohol-like odor, or show other signs of deterioration.

Meat/Poultry/Fish

1. Know your supplier; if possible, talk personally with the meat manager or butcher to find out which days fresh supplies are received and to probe their judgments about the freshness of various items. If you explain your concern, they may volunteer some helpful information—such as an opinion that farm-raised catfish arrives fresher than salmon from distant waters, for example.
2. Buy and use, or freeze, items well in advance of the expiration date on package.
3. Avoid any item with an off odor, unusual color, or surface slime.
4. In general, small cuts, such as ground meats or kabobs, deteriorate more quickly than larger cuts; the former definitely should be used or frozen in one or two days after purchasing.
5. Organ meats and seafood are particularly risky because they deteriorate at a much faster rate than other types of meat.
6. At home, rearrange packaging so that products can breathe, and store them in the coldest part of the refrigerator.

Breads/Pastries

Avoid if mold is visible on the product or anywhere in the package.

Cheese

Avoid visible mold; freeze if not eaten within a few days after opening.

Alcohol: Offender Extraordinaire

Not only the traditionally forbidden red wines, but ethanol itself, the defining chemical in any alcoholic beverage, is an extremely potent VAS and thus is to be avoided by the prudent sufferer. In addition to alcohol itself, alcoholic beverages contain a whole host of other migraine-provoking agents. These include natural sulfites, tyramine, and molds, all of which form during the fermentation process; supplementary sulfites, in many cases, added to speed this process; and phenols, chemicals in grape skins that are more prevalent in red wines. (Even though nonalcoholic beer obviously contains no ethanol, regrettably it does contain many of these other troublesome substances and so cannot be considered safe for migraineurs.) Congeners, too—substances that give each variety of liquor its distinctive flavor—are strongly suspected headache triggers. And as if this is not enough, a wide variety of potentially troublesome preservatives may be thrown into the vat during the manufacturing process as well.

In a susceptible person, any one of these ingredients alone can cause a headache, and so you can see why they have such destructive power, appearing as they do in combination in a typical drink. No alcoholic beverage can be considered safe for the migraineur. In the long-term, alcohol consumption seems to lower serotonin levels, thus contributing in a basic way to increased migraine susceptibility. Nonetheless, experts speculate about which forms of alcohol are the least harmful. The most frequent, although by no means unanimous, winners are vodka, gin, and white wine, preferably Riesling. *Tread lightly in this minefield, if at all.*

MSG: Potent and Pervasive

Adverse reactions to monosodium glutamate, and other forms of glutamate, are known to be widespread and exceptionally unpleasant. In a recent review of the health effects of this preservative, Dr. Alfred Scopp of the Northern California Headache Clinic believes that at least one third of migraineurs are sensitive to this substance. Some estimate the number to be even higher. The American Council for Headache Education (ACHE) suggests in its printed dietary guidelines that a significant number of migraineurs are able to eliminate attacks completely solely by avoiding this chemical. In fact, because MSG is such a potent vasodilator, virtually all migraine experts advocate its avoidance, a task that is much easier said than done in our present-day Western society.

It comes as a great surprise to most people that, under FDA regulations, manufacturers are not required candidly to list the MSG in their products as an ingredient on the labels. Currently, this chemical may be concealed under such terms as spice, natural flavoring, or simply flavoring or seasoning; when MSG occurs as part of another ingredient, it can appear as Kombu extract, sodium caseinate, hydrolyzed vegetable protein (or HVP), hydrolyzed plant protein, soy protein isolate, or simply vegetable protein.

It is no exaggeration to say that, at least in the 20th century United States, all commercially prepared foods should be suspect for MSG. Complicating our avoidance task is the fact that the additive really has no distinctive taste or appearance to give away its presence; as a rule of thumb, however, *if a dish tastes exceptionally salty, particular caution is in order.*

In this note only a few of the problem areas will be highlighted. You can find extremely comprehensive and helpful guidelines for tackling this difficult detective work in a book called *In Bad Taste: The MSG Syndrome,* by Santa Fe physician Dr. George Schwartz. This little jewel of a paperback, a "must read" for migraine sufferers and other MSG-sensitive people, was published in 1988 by Health Press; it is available in many public libraries throughout this country or can be purchased for a very modest price either through your local book store or directly from Health Press, PO Box 367, Santa Fe, NM 87501.

Of course the seasoning Accent is pure MSG; seasoning mixes—such as Lawry's Seasoned Salt, McCormick's Season All, Lemon Pepper, and Taco Seasoning—frequently contain hefty doses of this so-called flavor enhancer, as do cubed and powdered bouillon and most soups and gravies, whether mixes or canned varieties. Roasted nuts and chips, especially the flavored kind like barbecue or sour cream, often contain the chemical, as does much prebasted poultry and canned fish.

Dr. Schwartz points out the frightening fact that MSG is present not only in most packaged, canned, and frozen entrees in our supermarkets, but that it also is served to us frequently in the school lunch program, in restaurants—including, but certainly not limited to, fast-food establishments—and in airline meals as well. I always carry my own meals and snacks when flying. Avoiding this chemical in restaurant meals presents a special challenge since it often sneaks into the food in the guise of a seasoning salt or bouillon cube ingredient whose presence is honestly unknown to the cooks and other responsible personnel.

The safety of the new leaner ground beef products in which part of the fat has been replaced with other ingredients is very much in doubt. In the case of McDonald's version, the McLean Burger, the carrageenan filler is a likely MSG carrier (at any rate, it's a vegetable gum, high in dopamine); the bulk version of basically the same product, sold in supermarkets under various brand names, usually contains "beef flavoring," another likely MSG code word. My daughter was quite distressed to discover that she gets headaches after eating the McLean Burgers. I'm avoiding both versions like the plague.

For more specific MSG-avoidance strategies, see the notes later in this section under the topics of "Soy" (page 92) and "Restaurant Meals" (page 97).

Enough gloom; now for some sunshine. There are some MSG-free commercial products out there; we just have to look hard to find them. Canned tuna, for instance, whose label reads simply tuna and water, or tuna, water, and salt, can be assumed to be safe on this score. Star Kist calls such a chunk light product "diet tuna"; General Nutrition Center, the national health food chain, offers a comparable, though somewhat more expensive, product. As of this writing, the other major tuna canners are not marketing MSG-free products in my area; they probably will soon, however, in response to consumer backlash sure to follow the FDA's new labeling requirements, scheduled for May, 1994. (As of that date, products containing "significant and functional" levels of this chemical are to indicate its presence on the label, probably listed simply as glutamate.) Libby's canned salmon is MSG-free and usually of relatively high quality. Campbell's is now offering an MSG-free line of soups, called "Healthy Request"—truly a step forward for us migraineurs, although these soups still contain many rather mysterious chemicals and should be approached cautiously. My daughter and I have enjoyed the tomato without ill effect. (Evidently it contains very little tomato.) I sometimes use Swanson's canned reduced-sodium chicken broth, "Home-style" they call it; the manufacturer assures us that this product contains no MSG but seems uncertain about the presence of yeast flavoring. I proceed with caution, using it only in a pinch to extend insufficient portions of my honest-to-goodness homemade stock.

In the way of snacks, unflavored potato chips are usually safe (check the label) as are plain roasted nuts. Herr's makes a good "Slightly Salted" potato chip, which I can justify as an occasional treat. (The risks of excessive sodium and fat are discussed later.) I thoroughly enjoy Blue Diamond can-ned almonds, natural style, right off my supermarket shelf, and roasted sunflower seeds from the General Nutrition Center stores, mixing salted and unsalted varieties of the latter. (My hunch is that nuts and seeds might have acquired their bad rap because they frequently are flavored with MSG; these foods show up as forbidden fare on most migraine diets, but I have always eaten them cautiously, and to my heart's delight, I might add, without appar-ent ill effect. I especially appreciate nuts and seeds since I've had to give up many other quick and portable foods; these make a nice lunch, occasionally, along with a piece of fruit, either at home or when brown-bagging. (*See* cautions about nuts/seeds in the earlier section, "Challenging the Experts.")

The manufacturers of Mrs. Dash seasoning mixes assure us that all of their seasoning products are free of both MSG and yeast extracts. I also am delighted to be able to indulge in Bull's-Eye Barbecue Sauce, original style—apparently MSG free—for a big treat on my chicken.

Caffeine: The Paradox

The chemical caffeine occurs in many of our most beloved beverages, including coffee, tea, hot chocolate, most brown soft drinks (root beer is an exception), and some other sodas as well. Frequently it also appears in over-the-counter drugs, such as Anacin and Excedrin, as well as in many cold remedies. In migraineurs and others whose blood vessels are unstable, this chemical can cause a problem known as withdrawal headache. First, the chemical constricts the vessels, but as the body eliminates it, the vessels begin to expand and go into painful spasm. Typically, susceptible indivi-duals who ingest caffeine throughout the day feel fine as long as their supply continues uninterrupted, but they may wake up toward morning with a pain-ful headache. Such an occurrence is even more likely on weekends or any time such sensitive coffee drinkers sleep later than usual.

Just keep in mind the following facts about caffeine. A cup of brewed coffee can contain anywhere from 75 to 155 mg of caffeine, with drip coffee in the higher range and the percolated variety in the lower; the instant kind has considerably less, about 66 mg. The caffeine content of tea varies widely as well, both with the variety used and the brewing time: using a bag of black tea, a one-minute brew produces about 28 mg, whereas a three-minute brewing time results in about 44 mg. Please remember that all of these fig-ures (data supplied by the FDA) pertain to 5-oz cups—hardly the amount consumed by the typical person.

Colas and "pepper" drinks measure out at between 32 and 65 mg per 12-oz can, and surprisingly enough even some clear sodas contain hefty amounts of the chemical, with Mountain Dew and Mello Yello testing at slightly over 50 mg each. A half-ounce bar of sweet chocolate may contain as much as 10 mg of caffeine, and a cup of cocoa has about 5 mg. When figuring total caffeine consumption, don't forget to add amounts contained in some over-the-counter drugs: Check the labels on your pain relievers, weight-control aids, diuretics, and cold and allergy remedies, all of which may contain some caffeine.

Some migraine diets allow up to two 5-oz cups of coffee or tea a day, but the safest course is to swear off daily caffeine in any form. If you decide to decrease or eliminate the amount of this chemical you're ingesting to see whether your symptoms improve, you'd better do so gradually to minimize the likelihood of withdrawal headache.

Migraineurs can accomplish this weaning process in one of several ways: by decreasing the number of caffeine doses ingested throughout the day (for example, cutting back from four colas to three, and so on, over a period of a week or two until all have been eliminated); or by decreasing the amount of caffeine in each serving by substituting part of a decaffeinated beverage each time; or by some combination of these two methods. For example, a heavy coffee drinker might begin by switching from dripped coffee, which has the highest caffeine content, to the regular old-fashioned perked variety, and then finally to instant, which has the lowest caffeine content of all types. After that switch has been accomplished, the migraineur might then begin to replace a part of each cup of the instant beverage with a portion of decaf until completely weaned. Very heavy consumption of even decaffeinated beverages could possibly prove to be a problem for a highly sensitive migraineur. If you decide to cut down on your consumption of even purged beverages, replace them with some safe liquid in order to keep your juices flowing, so to speak. (Water, diluted apple or cranberry juice, 7-Up, low-fat milk, or weak herb tea [no ginseng] is probably safe for most of us, assuming the absence of personal allergy to any of those beverages.)

Restricting caffeine was the first migraine-related dietary change I made, and I was happy to receive a big payoff from it. Over a two week period, I gradually cut my daily coffee consumption from several cups of the strong perked variety to my current one cup of instant decaf. (I've never used caffeine-containing soft drinks or medication.) This change represented a major sacrifice; I was definitely dependent on that efficient chemical to open my eyes in the morning and to keep me alert during the day. My worst withdrawal symptoms—fatigue and irritability—were over after about three days of "being clean" at the end of the second week, though, and I've certainly never regretted my decision. Fortunately I did not experience increased headaches as part of the withdrawal process.

The paradox is this: In the short term, caffeine can help to halt a migraine attack if it is taken early enough; in the long term, however, the chemical usually worsens our disorder because of the rebound action described above. Beware! It may make sense for some sufferers to use this chemical to halt an attack, but the wisdom of its use as a daily beverage has been sharply called into question.

Cured/Canned Meats: Definite "No, Nos"

Canned and cured meats represent a triple threat. First, freshness of ingredients cannot be assumed, particularly in cured meats, where aging is part of the manufacturing process. Second, nitrites, MSG, and other chemical triggers are common ingredients. Third, many of these products are high in saturated fats. I avoid all of these items like the plague, with few exceptions—one canned meat and two canned fish products—that seem to avoid the risks outlined above and to be relatively tasty and convenient as well. Gerber's chicken and meat sticks (baby food packed in glass jars) and some varieties of canned salmon (Libby's) and tuna (Chicken of the Sea diet pack) are MSG-free and apparently of fresh quality. Because freshness can't be guaranteed in canned meat and fish, however, Level III people or extremely cautious Level II adherents would be taking some risk with these products. For several years, I avoided canned fish entirely; now I eat it occasionally, sometimes experiencing adverse reactions (presumably because of the high histamine content of cold-water fish).

Soy: It Sneaks, Then Socks

Soy derivatives, which are very high in dopamine, can easily wind up in our diets—invisible but wreaking painful consequences. They are included in a wide variety of products ranging from vegetarian entrees, such as veggie burgers and other meat twins like artificial bacon bits (Baco's and other brands, often on salad bars), to cream soups, and bread and pastry products such as donuts, sweet rolls, English muffins, and dessert sponge cakes.

Some products will honestly admit the derivative; soy flour, for example, often is plainly listed on labels of baked goods and prepared mixes. (I now use Aunt Jemima's Buckwheat Pancake Mix instead of my previous whole wheat selection by the same manufacturer, so as to avoid the soy flour in the latter.) Soups and meat substitutes may designate a soy ingredient simply as vegetable protein. These soy proteins often contain natural MSG as well, thus delivering double trouble. This is another case in which informed and careful label reading is absolutely essential.

Soy sauce, an obvious source of both soy and MSG, is a potent trigger. The safety of soy lecithin—often listed simply as lecithin—is in question, but because it usually appears in baked goods in very small amounts, it's unlikely to represent much of a problem. Use of lecithin supplements, some-times sold in health food stores as an Alzheimer's preventive, is probably unwise for migraineurs, however. Soybean oil, an ingredient in many com-mercial baked goods and salad dressings, on the other hand, is perfectly safe; the oil is highly refined and does not contain any of the dopamine present in other forms of soy.

It's regrettable that such a nutritious food as soy frequently causes not only headaches but various allergic reactions as well. Health-conscious con-sumers may be at a greater risk of getting into trouble with this ingredient than the average person, who probably wouldn't be caught dead eating a veggie burger. Tofu, the highly nutritious soybean product so popular in Oriental dishes, is forbidden food for migraineurs, as is misu, another soy-based Oriental favorite, used as a soup ingredient. Likewise, we must shun soy-based ice cream substitutes. Soy-containing diet shakes and bars, which form the basis for virtually all prepackaged commercial weight-loss pro-grams, can rapidly cause a migraine crisis as well. The only soy-free prod-uct of this type offered by either drug or health-food stores in my area contains a yeast extract and therefore poses an equally powerful threat. Two of my acquaintances trace the beginning of their painful episodes to the use of these meal-replacement products.

Salad Dressing and Condiments: Chemistry 101

Chemicals in most commercial salad dressings and condiments pose an unacceptable risk to migraine sufferers, at least if ingested in large quanti-ties. MSG and sulfites are standard fare; other undesirable ingredients are variety vinegars (only white distilled is safe) and various gum derivatives used as thickeners (these members of the legume family should be avoided). Unless you are taking a very strict approach, however, an occasional indulgence in one of these potions probably will do no harm. Just indulge sparingly. In restaurants, ordering the dressing on the side makes sense.

For regular home use, I use instead a mixture of three parts of distilled white vinegar (diluted with water if taste dictates) and one part of any preferred vegetable oil. (I like a good olive.) To this mixture I add small amount of sugar and garlic powder. Then I liberally sprinkle dressed salads with any desired herb; my favorites are oregano or basil, but sometimes dill provides a pleasant change.

If you are lucky and read labels carefully, you can probably find a relatively pure local brand of mayo-type (but lower in fat than the real thing) salad dressing. That product can be safely used as a sandwich spread or diluted with vinegar, sugar, and water to make a creamy-type dressing for salads. Celery seed makes a nice addition in lieu of herbs.

Condiments such as steak sauce, mustard, ketchup, and horseradish may be based on undistilled vinegar containing tyramine, and may contain troublesome preservatives as well; they need to be approached with the same caution as do salad dressings. Occasional picking may be okay, while pigging-out can lead to trouble.

Vitamin–Mineral Supplementation: A Mixed Bag

There is little conclusive evidence linking either a deficiency or excess of vitamins and minerals to headaches. The most clear-cut studies in this regard show that too much Vitamin A can cause or worsen symptoms. On the other hand, research points to a possible benefit from Vitamin E supplementation; this vitamin apparently decreases platelet stickiness thought to contribute to migraine—the same action performed by the now popular daily aspirin. In addition, some biochemists note the requirement for an ample supply of certain B vitamins in the enzyme actions that breakdown dietary amines, indicating a possible advantage for migraineurs in Vitamin B supplementation. Finally, recent preliminary studies suggest a correlation, although not necessarily a cause and effect relationship, between magnesium deficiency and migraine. (Scientists don't know which causes which, but the two conditions often occur together.)

I personally take daily supplements of B-complex (15 mg), Vitamin E (200 mg), and Magnesium (500 mg). These are not considered massive doses. My supplements are all nonallergenic—yeast and preservative free— properties that make sense for anyone with allergic tendencies, especially for migraineurs.

During several periods when I was taking massive doses of Vitamin C (3–4 grams a day) to prevent recurrence of a bladder infection, I noticed a significant worsening of my migraine symptoms. I now take less than one gram of Vitamin C each day, based strictly on that negative personal experience. I have been unable to find any reference to Vitamin C in the headache literature, one way or the other, but taking relatively low levels of this vitamin makes sense as a way to replace sacrificed citrus. Be especially cautious if you use this supplement while on an antidepressant, however. The medical literature indicates that the vitamin actually decreases the effectiveness of those medications.

Restricting Fat: A Prudent Regimen

Evidence suggests that excessive amounts of certain types of dietary fat may worsen migraine. Both controlled studies and the self-reports of sufferers suggest the substance as a possible headache provoker. At least in the long-term, a diet high in animal fats and/or hydrogenated vegetable oils increases the tendency of blood cells called platelets to clump together; and many experts believe that this platelet stickiness worsens any existing migraine tendencies.

Many of the changes already mentioned will result in overall reduction of saturated fat. For instance, avoiding cured meat and hard cheese will automatically decrease fat consumption. A few additional precautions, such as choosing lean cuts of meat—such as beef round or flank, white meat of poultry, and occasional pork tenderloin—will help too. Trimming all fat from meat, baking or broiling instead of frying, minimizing the use of ground beef, discarding poultry skin, using only low-fat dairy products, and eating two fish meals a week (if you're lucky enough to find a "fresh" supply) should put you well on your way to a prudent diet—not only from the standpoint of migraine control, but from a general good-health perspective as well. Limiting yourself to two or three eggs a week and avoiding mayonnaise make sense too. In baking, and even when making scrambled egg dishes, egg whites can usually be substituted for at least part of the whole eggs called for, without sacrificing quality. The commercially prepared low-fat egg products seem unwise for migraineurs—some contain MSG and/or mystery ingredients.

Avoiding tropical and hydrogenated vegetable oils presents a bit more of a challenge. Cookie and cracker manufacturers who have been scurrying to delete tropical oils from their products tend to replace them with the hydrogenated variety—hardly an improvement, if the truth be told. Just go very easy on such products—no bingeing on commercial cookies and potato chips. Pretzels are an acceptable snack in this regard, but many varieties are excessively salty and may contain malt.

Excessive Sodium: The Clouds Gather

Recent evidence suggests that too much sodium contributes to platelet clumping, a tendency thought to aggravate migraine. This finding supports a suspicion long held by some researchers and sufferers that salt can act as a migraine trigger. Thus far, however, no controlled studies conclusively forge this link.

Most of the sodium we consume is not in the form of table salt, but rather as additives in processed foods. To minimize sodium consumption, carefully read labels, watching for all forms of sodium, and build menus around nonprocessed or lightly processed foods. Manufacturers seem to be getting the message that Americans want to reduce sodium intake, and more and more lower salt alternatives are becoming available. As was true with fats, many of the dietary changes already suggested will result in a reduction in sodium.

Coping Strategies for the Steady Customer

If, during a conscientious trial, you notice an improvement in your symptoms and decide to continue to follow one of the three levels of the VAS Total Load Approach, you will face an interesting challenge. Here are some possible ways to maximize your chances for successful adherence while minimizing the feeling of deprivation that often goes along with restrictive diets.

Practical Tips: Accentuating the Positive

Creating New Recipes

Armed with a list of foods you can safely eat, adapt some old favorite recipes by making substitutions or create new dishes to replace those you must give up. You might want to ask a creative friend or even a registered dietitian to lend a hand.

In Appendix E are the results of some of my culinary adaptations and creations; these particular dishes may not excite your taste buds, but at least they will give you some idea about what can be done. Overall, I use more herbs and spices in my cooking now, including moderate amounts of both onion and garlic powder to replace those forbidden whole ingredients; this substitution works well and causes me no apparent problems, although I can't explain why. I also eat more green and red bell peppers along with radishes to replace the zing lost from sacrificing onion in salads. I use lots of brown rice and cottage cheese; the latter can be blended to create dips, with cucumber and dill, or paprika, and can also substitute for sour cream or yogurt, both on baked potatoes and in certain casseroles.

Sometimes I sneak small amounts of tomato juice into soups (It's surprising the good effect just a little of this can have.) I also love the taste of chopped apples and bananas gently tossed in a mixture of orange and pineapple juice (I pour off the juice before eating and just enjoy the residual citrus flavor). When I get a hot dog craving, I slice several Gerber's meat sticks on a bun with a little mustard, and I'm in business. Pretty tasty when split, browned under the broiler and served with pancakes too. This product offers the added advantage of being conveniently packaged and therefore handy for brown bagging.

Helpful Products: A Personal Discovery

In my personal quest for safe foods to replace the eliminated items, the following products (some of which may not be available in all sections of the country) have been a godsend:

Aunt Jemima Buckwheat Pancake Mix (no soy)
Breyers' Ice Milk: vanilla, butter pecan, and almond (no vegetable gums)
Bull's-Eye Original Style Barbecue Sauce (No MSG)
Campbell's Healthy Request Soups (no MSG), varieties appropriate to level
Del Monte Snack Cups: Vanilla Pudding (no vegetable gums)
Gerber's Meat Sticks (no MSG or sulfites; fresh quality)
Herr's Slightly Salted Potato Chips (no MSG)
Mrs. Dash Seasoning
Nabisco Shredded Wheat (no added bran or malt)
Popeye Puffed Wheat (no added malt or gums)

Restaurant Meals: A Rocky Road

Eating out safely is a challenging experience at best. Whenever possible, try to patronize only a few familiar restaurants, especially when first starting your dietary management program. Your diary entries should tell you whether the meals there are contributing to your symptoms. Keep these points in mind before ordering:

1. Ask for assurance that fish or meat is fresh or fresh-frozen (without preservatives). Consider daily specials; items tend to be fresher when turnover is high.
2. Ask about the presence of MSG in breaded meat/fish, or avoid coating entirely for complete safety.
3. Avoid soups and gravies since they almost always contain large amounts of MSG.

4. Request that no mixed seasonings be used on your foods; many contain MSG.
5. Avoid meat tenderizers and marinades; the former usually are papaya based, the latter made from soy or teriyaki sauces.
6. If considering shellfish, ask whether sulfites have been added, not in the restaurant, but by the supplier or shipper. To be sure, someone will have to check the shipping carton.
7. Order salad dressings on the side or ask for distilled vinegar and oil.
8. Ask whether breads and pastries are made from a mix. If so, they may contain soy flour; someone will have to check the label to be sure. Items made from scratch are usually safe if not sourdough.
9. On the salad bar, avoid pickled dishes, especially meat and fish.

Since addressing your concerns will require the staff's attention, it is usually better if you telephone ahead at a slack time and cover some of these points with a chef or manager. You are apt to receive more accurate information and meet less resentment by following that course.

If you are fighting severe symptoms, and circumstances force you to eat in an unfamiliar restaurant, you usually can get a safe meal by ordering a fresh salad (no onion or tomato), broiled steak or chicken (no tenderizer, marinade or seasoning salt), and baked potato. In cafeterias when nothing else seems safe, I select fried chicken and then remove the skin before eating. Steak-house chains may be especially difficult. So many of their meats contain either tenderizers or marinades that ground beef is often the only safe choice.

Not Offending Perle Mesta: A Personal Challenge

The experience of eating in someone's private home can be even more difficult than eating in a restaurant, especially if the hostess is not a close personal friend who can be questioned closely and expected to cooperate without resentment. You may feel more comfortable eating ahead of time and just picking cautiously from a buffet table. Of course such an "eat and pick" strategy is harder to pull off in the setting of a sit-down dinner party, although if you try it you may be surprised to learn how little other guests notice what you do or do not eat. In any case, the best rule of thumb is to avoid soups, gravies, cured and breaded meats, and pickled dishes. Steer clear of exceptionally salty items. Again, your safest bets are unadorned poultry, vegetables, and fruits not noted as risky in the previous chapter.

Outwitting the Unknown

If you can foresee being in a mealtime setting where you may be confronted with foods of unknown quality, plan ahead either by eating first or by taking a snack along. Then if it turns out that you are offered some safe foods after all, you will be free to exercise your options without the pressure of a growling stomach and falling blood sugar. Examples of such scenarios include airline meals, unfamiliar restaurants, or catered parties.

Psychological Tricks

Self-Talk

In a broader sense, I have successfully battled deprivation by using a little positive self-talk. During one emotionally low period, I posted the following sign in my kitchen as a reminder that things could be worse: "It is not a tragedy that Susan cannot eat certain foods." At least I chuckled occasionally when I read it, and it became quite a conversation piece. Another example of positive self-talk: I listed all the things readily coming to mind for which I continue to be thankful; the resulting pages reassured me that, in spite of my many sacrifices, much that is good and pleasurable remains in my life. Any time I feel particularly negative, I usually can turn myself around quickly by retreating behind closed doors and reading this list aloud.

Knowing Our Response: Satisfied or Stimulated?

When you're feeling generally deprived or have an overpowering food craving, it helps to know how you react to tasting. Does sampling a desired food satisfy you and stop your "obsessing" over it, or does just one taste usually create an urge for another, possibly leading to a binge? Plan your strategy in accordance with your reaction. I'm grateful that I'm primarily a satisfied taster; I can have just one bite of my husband's lasagna, for example, and then forget about it. On the other hand, I don't want to be anywhere near pizza or pizza-eaters.

If you know you can't handle tasting, then don't indulge. If sights and smells are too tempting, then remove yourself from them or them from you, if possible. There's no point in torturing yourself unnecessarily. If preparing personally forbidden foods for others is a miserable experience, then you don't have to do it. It's probably not fair to ask intimates to follow your diet either, though. Strike some compromises.

I feel comfortable accompanying my family to a German restaurant where virtually no MSG-free dishes are served, because the staff knows us well and has no objection to my occupying a chair and nibbling on carrot sticks from home. On the other hand, I resoundingly refused a similar invitation to eat at a pizza place because watching others enjoy that favorite dish would bring me nothing but misery. Knowing how I'm likely to react to specific situations helps me to keep on the right dietary track with a minimum of pain.

Grieving Over Our Losses

At times when I find myself missing some favorite food and feeling especially deprived and pitiful, I grab a pen and paper and write out a journal entry describing my feelings in a very detailed and somewhat dramatic way. I use this same technique to get any disturbing feeling, such as anger or frustration, off my chest when it seems to be interfering with my ability to concentrate.

The Good News: *Dietary Changes Bring Improvement*

I am convinced that many sufferers can improve significantly by changing their diets in varying degrees. As a very informal experiment, I surveyed the readers who helped me with this book to see whether they had put any of the dietary suggestions they had read about into practice and, if so, to what result. Not all read the entire book, and so some are not even familiar with the dietary chapters. It was quite heartening to learn that two readers who worked on the diet chapters had made serious efforts to integrate the material into their own lives. As a result one person was not only able to stop preventive medication, but even managed to decrease attacks from one every few weeks to one every few months; the other, a less severe sufferer, stopped having painful attacks altogether through a combination of dietary change and the use of ibuprofen to interrupt symptoms when they first appear.

The Big Picture: *Principles of Effective Dietary Management*

1. Only your doctor and/or a registered dietitian can provide complete and definitive information about personal nutritional requirements.
2. To avoid tyramine:
   a. Eat only the highest quality food; reject any that has begun to deteriorate. Fish and organ meats deteriorate quickly, as does certain produce, such as strawberries, raspberries, spinach, and leaf lettuce.
   b. Avoid anything fermented, dried, pickled or otherwise aged (except fresh items pickled at home in distilled vinegar).
   c. Choose frozen fish and vegetables (plain) over canned products, often even over so-called fresh ones, if freshness is in doubt.
   d. Be leery of anything whose freshness cannot be verified visually, such as canned juices, applesauce, or frozen greens, for example.
   e. Minimize products made with yeast; avoid yeast extracts.

3. Avoid or restrict consumption of:

Alcohol	Aspartame (Equal™)
Chocolate	Nitrites

Other foods
   naturally high in amines
   and phenols
	Sulfites

Caffeine	Food colorings
Monosodium glutamate (MSG)	Benzoate

4. Follow a diet low in saturated and hydrogenated fats and relatively low in sodium.
5. Strictly follow these recommendations for at least six weeks to test your susceptibility to dietary triggers.
6. Keep a food diary (either daily or periodically) during that six-week period and evaluate patterns weekly.

Balance to Be Achieved

To enjoy tasty, nutritious, emotionally satisfying food while avoiding, or at least minimizing, migraine symptoms.

Chapter 7

The Risk of Femininity

Turning Lemons into Lemonade

Female Majority: *Whys and Wherefores*

Whether or not you put any stock in the biblical account of Eve's punishment in the Garden of Eden, it's hard not to notice that migraine is primarily an affliction of women. Experts estimate that about three out of four migraine sufferers are female. Because this feminine domination of the disorder emerges only after puberty, and the occurrence of migraines waxes and wanes dramatically along with changes in the female reproductive cycle, it seems obvious that a powerful interaction is taking place between the migraine process and fluctuating female hormones. Experts recognize that sex hormones directly affect the central nervous system, the site where migraine seems to have its roots. In fact, it is no exaggeration to say that the single most important migraine influence in women is hormonal. For the individual female sufferer, this means that the first place to start looking for an explanation of worsening symptoms is in a changing hormone balance. And more often than not, it is we migraineurs, rather than our doctors, who must be the vigilant ones in such situations.

Considering the importance of this interaction between female hormones and migraine, relatively little controlled research has been done on the subject, and many gynecologists continue to ignore decades-old data showing that migraineurs fare far better on noncyclical rather than cyclical supplements. Perhaps this neglect is yet another example of how women's health concerns have been minimized.

For many years, women have noticed that the frequency and severity of their headaches are linked to certain hormone fluctuations, with increased symptoms usually occurring shortly before or during their periods. There seems to be a small group of women for whom menstruation is their only trigger—that is, they experience attacks *only* during or shortly before their periods. For most women, however, menstruation seems to lower the migraine threshold—that is, although they may well experience attacks during other times of the month, they have more frequent and more severe attacks just before or during their periods. Trigger exposures that would not set off attacks at other times do so with a vengeance then. Additionally, many women have observed that attacks decrease or disappear entirely during the last six months of pregnancy, especially if headaches were associated with menstrual periods. Postpartum headaches (headaches occurring right after or within a few days of giving birth) are quite common, particularly in women with a migraine history. In some women headaches do not resume until ovulation begins again, sometimes when breastfeeding is discontinued.

Looking at the broader picture of life-span changes, some women cite a dramatic increase in symptoms during the premenopausal and menopausal years, whereas others notice a gradual decrease at about this same time. Traditional thinking holds that symptoms gradually decrease with age in both men and women, but at least one recent study challenges that belief. (Of course, men have sex hormones too, but their levels are relatively stable, not disturbed by the frequent fluctuations occurring in women.)

The popularity of oral contraceptives called dramatic attention to this long-observed relationship between female hormones and migraine. Many women noted a significant change in previous symptoms in relationship to the "pill"—whether for good or ill—and others first experienced attacks after beginning the hormones. Usually, if symptoms worsen after starting oral contraception, headaches are most common during the days after estrogen has been stopped. For many years, experts assumed that the estrogen content in itself was responsible for the often worsening migraine symptoms associated with the pill, but this conclusion is not really consistent with what we know about the relationship between migraine and naturally occurring hormone changes. The times when women report the greatest headache susceptibility are times when their estrogen levels are either low or falling. This connection between falling estrogen levels and increased migraine vulnerability was first documented in 1972, but for some reason the suspected link was largely ignored for nearly two decades.

Some researchers are finally beginning to offer a more logical explanation of the relationship between female hormones and migraine. For example, British migraine authority Dr. M. K. Ghose, writing in 1984, explains his finding that female migraineurs are more vulnerable to the known dietary trigger tyramine in weeks four and one of their cycles—that is, just before and during menses, when estrogen levels are low—than they are in midcycle when the hormone is at its height. To avoid this apparently troublesome estrogen dip, some migraine specialists now advocate use of the estrogen patch for women who experience severe premenstrual migraines that don't improve with other treatment.

In older migraineurs who need ongoing estrogen supplements to prevent hot flashes or the risk of osteoporosis, this patch appears to be the best way to go. The key to successful supplementation seems to be maintaining a relatively low but constant level of estrogen, avoiding the sudden drops that may occur either naturally or with the common cyclical dosage that calls for cutting down and/or stopping estrogen when progesterone is begun.

Some studies show that in many women oral contraceptives either initiate migraine episodes or worsen already existing symptoms. This tendency for the pill to worsen migraine seems to hold true for many sufferers even when they use the lower-dose estrogen contraceptives available in the 1990s. Medical opinion is firmly against oral contraceptive use in those women whose headaches are either initiated or worsened by the hormones: In fact, there is a fear that continued use of the pill under those circumstances may actually increase the risk of stroke, a risk that, as studies now show, is already relatively high in migraineurs. Researchers continue to look into this possible pill–stroke link, but if you don't like to gamble with your health, perhaps you would rather err on the side of safety until more definite information is available.

One further word of caution here: In most migraineurs who have experienced either initial or worsening symptoms while on the pill, symptoms return to their prepill level within a few months after use stops; for a small number of these women, however, increased symptoms, once having been set in motion by the hormones, will continue. Migraineurs may be better served by choosing a different form of contraception and certainly should always level with their doctors about headache symptoms when discussing contraceptive choices.

The following sections discuss some possible ways of dealing with hormone related symptoms—or, in other words, ways that will help you turn your lemons into lemonade.

Knowing Your Lemons: *Keep a Diary*

This subject keeps popping up in various chapters for a very good reason—it's extremely important. You may want to review what Chapters 3 and 5 have to say about keeping a headache diary to track triggers and threshold-setters. And remember the sample format provided in Appendix A. Of course, as this chapter emphasizes, hormone changes are the biggest single threshold-setter for women, and so in order to be helpful, your headache

diary must note the day of your menstrual cycle and information about hormone supplements along with any other data recorded about symptoms, suspected triggers, and so on.

If you are a woman between puberty and menopause, you probably know
that the first day of your period should be counted as day number one each
cycle. But if you have irregular cycles, then you may not be able to rely
simply on the day of the month to predict when your time of increased vulnerability will come again. Your body will, however, give you some signs
when it ovulates, and even women with very irregular cycles will probably
find that the time between ovulation and menstruation is predictable. Often
a change in cervical mucous is one clue that ovulation is about to take place.
Usually at about midcycle the mucus becomes more profuse and also
stringier. In most women, a period will follow within about 14–16 days.

However you are able to determine it, try to be aware of the day of your
cycle in relation to your headache symptoms. By charting both in your
diary, soon you may be able to see a pattern. The most common time of
increased headache susceptibility is, as already stated, just before, during,
or immediately after your period, but a few women experience more
problems in the middle of their cycles. The point is to identify your own
problem phase, if any, and then to be especially careful to avoid triggers
and/or take preventive medications shortly before that phase is due to
occur the next time.

If you have entered menopause and are no longer having periods, you
may not be aware that you will probably continue to experience significant
hormone fluctuations for a number of years—hormonal ups and downs that
still can make you more vulnerable to migraine at certain times than others.
Therefore, even after menopause, reading your body's signals and noting
the specific day of your cycle in diary entries remains quite helpful. Obviously, maintaining such an awareness is harder when there is no menstrual
bleeding to guide you, but it can be developed nevertheless. Especially if
you regularly experienced premenstrual symptoms during your childbearing
years, you probably will be able to identify clues that it's that time of month.

If you haven't noticed such signals, try to be on the lookout for them. As
a postmenopausal woman myself, I notice that not only am I unusually tired
and slightly irritable for about four days out of each month, but that
I have extremely cold feet and slightly stiff joints during that "premenstrual" phase as well. In my own case, a lower migraine threshold or greater
headache vulnerability definitely accompanies those other premenstrual
symptoms during that four-day phase. The onset of those nonheadache
symptoms—the fatigue, irritability, cold feet, and stiff joints—serves as my
warning to be extra careful about avoiding triggers for the next few days.

After those typically preperiod symptoms pass, I then consider the next day as day number one of my cycle for the purposes of my headache diary.

Hormone Adustments: *Basic Threshold-Setters*

It is highly unlikely that hormone treatment will help women whose attacks are in no way related to menstruation. (An exception involves testosterone, a male hormone also present in women, that is discussed in a later section of this chapter.) But for most of us female sufferers who find that we are more susceptible to attacks during specific times of our menstrual cycles, certain hormone manipulations may make a world of difference in our migraine symptoms. We are indebted to Dr. Stephen D. Silberstein and Dr. George R. Merriam for taking a special interest in the migraine–hormone link and presenting a comprehensive outline of this most important subject in the June, 1991 issue of *Neurology*. The specific suggestions in the remainder of this chapter rely heavily on the work of these authorities.

Estrogen

Knowing that the most severe migraine symptoms tend to occur when estrogen levels fall is very helpful information. Some doctors will prescribe an estrogen supplement—given either orally or by means of a skin patch—to prevent that troublesome dip and thus forestall symptoms. Such estrogen supplements can be used on an occasional preventive basis in menstruating women without causing them to delay or miss a period. Women using hormone replacement therapy (HRT) after menopause or hysterectomy may want to adjust their estrogen supplements to work with their bodies' natural estrogen supplies in order to avoid such an anticipated dip. For example, one might change the patch slightly less often when natural estrogen supply is high (usually right after midcycle) and more often as natural supplies fall during the symptomatic phase discussed above.

Women using HRT sometimes find themselves in an uncomfortable bind: Migraine symptoms begin or are worsened by the hormones, but these individuals are in dire need of these supplements to prevent other problems. Such women should consider several possible alternatives: either lowering estrogen dose, changing the form of estrogen they take, and/or changing the method of administering the hormone. Doctors usually start women on oral estrogen rather than the patch, and the most common variety given seems to be the conjugated form. A woman who is having increased migraine symptoms on such a regimen might first try lowering her dose. If this move does not relieve her symptoms, she might try another form of the hormone—

either estradiol, synthetic estrogen, or pure estrone. She also may wish to consider varying her dose during her cycle, as suggested above, to work with her body's own natural supply. One preliminary study found that postmenopausal women could solve this dilemma by switching from oral dosage to the skin patch and by adding testosterone (sometimes called androgen) to their supplements.

In addition to allowing women to maintain a low but even estrogen level, the patch has another advantage over oral dosing for migraineurs. Some hormone experts point out that because this transdermal supplementation avoids the first pass through the liver that occurs with oral administration, it fails to stimulate the clotting mechanism—an action much better done without in migraineurs who may already experience sticky platelets and an increased stroke risk. In spite of all the pluses offered by the patch, some women with super sensitive skin and/or allergic tendencies find that they are unable to tolerate it because of skin irritation, especially in hot weather. According to the manufacturer, sometimes such irritation can be avoided, or at least minimized, by wearing the patch on the buttocks, rather than on more sensitive areas of the trunk; and the drier the skin under the patch remains, the less likely irritation is to occur.

Progesterone

Progesterone levels don't appear to be critically related to migraine symptoms to the extent that estrogen levels are. If you are postmenopausal and receiving HRT, you will be required to take this hormone along with estrogen in order to avoid increased risk of uterine cancer. There are several ways progesterone can be taken, none of which have been shown to affect headache. A continuous low-dose administration of this hormone is probably best, however, since as a general rule migraineurs' bodies seem to prefer staying on an even keel.

Testosterone

Preliminary studies suggest that a decrease in the male hormone testosterone, which also is present in women (although in smaller amounts than in men), may play a crucial role in worsening migraine in some premenopausal and menopausal women. In fact the significance of decreased testosterone levels was recognized several decades ago, when researchers actually gave testosterone supplements to female subjects in controlled trials and were able to reduce their migraine symptoms significantly. Because very large doses of the male hormone were given, however, the women involved in this research developed superficial masculine characteristics, such as body-hair growth and deepening voices. These characteristics were judged unacceptable and possibly irreversible, and for that reason this valuable avenue of migraine research was abandoned.

In normal women, of course, testosterone does not produce masculine characteristics because it is kept in check by relatively larger amounts of female hormones. We now know that such undesirable side effects can be avoided completely by limiting the daily testosterone dose to ten milligrams or less—a level of supplementation now recommended by some gynecologists as a part of HRT in postmenopausal women. Testosterone also often increases lagging sexual interest and response, as well as relieving the somewhat more subtle, but still devastating, symptoms of fatigue and depression that frequently show up after menopause and often are not helped by estrogen alone.

In a recent Belgian study in which the hormone status of postmenopausal migraineurs was carefully evaluated, only one significant difference was found between the sufferers and a normal control group: The testosterone level of the migraine sufferers was significantly lower than that of the other women. However, those preliminary results must be repeated and evaluated before the medical community will consider acting further on them.

It is interesting to note that falling testosterone levels in animals are associated with a decrease in one of the enzymes that breaks down amines and that is thought to be deficient in migraineurs. Those findings suggest the importance of maintaining normal testosterone levels as a means of keeping migraine symptoms in check. If you happen to be a female around the age of menopause and have experienced the onset or worsening of migraine symptoms, I strongly encourage you to discuss testosterone supplementation with your doctor. The hormone may be particularly appropriate if you notice other symptoms of testosterone deficiency—signs such as dry skin, lagging sexual interest and/or response, fatigue, and mild depression that can't be explained by such other medical conditions as low thyroid hormone levels, anemia, or estrogen deficiency. Pay attention to these symptoms—they may be signals of a testosterone shortage just as hot flashes often are signs that you could benefit from added estrogen. What is helpful for these other symptoms certainly holds out a hope of helping your migraines as well.

Theory Versus Practice

There seem to be at least two important gaps between medical theory and practice regarding hormone supplementation. First, most hormone experts emphasize that the best level of hormone supplementation is the *lowest* one that will bring symptoms under reasonable control. In practice, unfortunately, little effort seems to go into helping women recognize that lowest effective level. Second, it is regrettable that very few practicing physicians, including neurologists and gynecologists, seem to be up-to-date on the best use of hormone supplements in relieving migraine. If you want to benefit from this research, you may need to lead your doctor gently. If you are reluctant to pursue this somewhat innovative course, then you may be faced with another decade of suffering while researchers conduct more studies and physicians become familiar with the ones already completed. Do you want lemons or lemonade?

Strong Medicine for Stubborn Cases

The first line of medical defense against premenstrual and menstrual migraine are nonsteroidal anti-inflammatory medications, such as naproxen sodium (Anaprox or the over-the-counter Aleve), meclofenamate (Meclomen), or mefenamic acid (Ponstel), on a regular basis for a few days to a week out of each month, as needed. This treatment is thought to be particularly appropriate because menstrual migraines frequently go hand-in-hand with cramps. Both of these conditions probably signal a surplus of inflammatory chemicals called prostaglandins. Sometimes the antihistamine cyproheptadine (Periactin) is used in the same way, as a periodic preventive at vulnerable times of the cycle.

In many cases, popular preventives—taken either in the traditional fashion or only during the most vulnerable time each month—are effective in combating menstrual migraines. Several people I know find relief from menstrual migraine by using low-level antidepressant medication all month and then increasing the dose a few days before their period is due; after the period ends, they return to the lower dose.

Unfortunately, hormone-driven attacks are among the most severe and treatment-resistant of all migraines. Sometimes ordinary preventives (discussed in Chapter 10) are unsuccessful in stopping these attacks. However, other medical approaches are available for menstrual migraines that fail to respond to trigger avoidance, hormone manipulation, the NSAIDs, Periactin, or common preventives. Sometimes ergot preparations, steroids, or major tranquilizers are used on a regular, but temporary, basis for up to a week each month, without a great risk of developing resistance or dependency.

Research shows that three other drugs—the synthetic androgen preparation, danazol; the dopamine agonist and prolactin blocker, bromocriptine (Parlodel); and the estrogen blocker, tamoxifen—can often be used to prevent particularly severe and stubborn menstrual migraines. These are potent drugs, however, as the subtitle above indicates, and they often cause very bothersome side effects. Danazol, for example, a drug that prevents normal bimonthly estrogen-level increases, and thus avoids the treacherous dips as well, often causes uncomfortable fluid retention and must be accompanied by a diuretic. Some women also experience hot flashes from it. Tamoxifen, too, dampens estrogen production, thus preventing sudden drops that are known to trigger migraines, and can cause hot flashes. On the other hand, one of these drugs, bromocriptine (Parlodel) has been shown to relieve other unpleasant premenstrual symptoms in some women in addition to helping hormone-driven headaches. This drug, too, causes troublesome side effects for some patients, including lightheadedness, nausea, and even headache. It can also lead to dry mouth, drowsiness, leg cramps, and loss of appetite.

Useful Information: Hormones, Men, and Doctors

It's important to know that treatments that change hormone levels sometimes relieve headache in men too—suggesting that some male migraineurs also might be suffering from a hormone imbalance. Pharmacologist Joe Graedon reports that a man who was experiencing decreased interest in sex, along with fatigue, low-level depression, and headache, responded very favorably to treatment with Parlodel. (Such men sometimes have difficulty achieving or maintaining erections and may have enlarged breasts.) And in a recent medical journal, a physician describes his serendipitous discovery that one male patient's migraines were significantly relieved by the use of the drug clomiphene, which originally had been prescribed to boost his low sperm count. (But rather ironically, that very same drug, usually sold as Clomid or Serophene and often used as a female fertility drug, sometimes is charged with causing headache in women.)

There are so many individual variations in this hormone–migraine link that general rules are hard to come by. Sometimes hormone-level measurements can provide a good starting point, but only individual trials can determine finally whether any of these potent hormone adjusters will relieve particular hormone-driven headache symptoms and, if so, whether their benefits will outweigh their possible downsides. A gynecologist with special interest in migraine would be the ideal doctor for female sufferers to consult if they wish to try one of these drugs. Male sufferers would need to see a urologist or an endocrinologist to determine whether or not a hormone imbalance might be contributing to symptoms. (A sperm count might not be a bad place to start in investigating such a possibility.)

Pregnancy: *Prepare Mom First, Then the Nursery*

Because few medications are permitted during pregnancy, out of concern for the developing baby, it's important for the migraineur who is anticipating motherhood to take some special steps. Quite often, natural relief from headache symptoms occurs after about the first three months of pregnancy. Unfortunately, however, during that early period when many women continue to experience attacks, drugs are considered to be the greatest danger to the fetus. Migraine authorities express particular concern about potential problems posed by fetal exposure to beta-blockers, ergot, and caffeine.

Moms-to-be can prepare themselves to get through what may be a difficult few months by making the effort to master biofeedback or other relaxation skills before becoming pregnant. Other helpful strategies include beginning a conscientious diary to identify triggers and making a trial run on a restrictive dietary program—both well in advance of the actual pregnancy, if at all possible. If you decide to nurse your baby and wish to continue avoiding medication as much as possible, these same strategies should remain helpful.

My Search For That Delicate Balance: *Trial, Error, and Success*

During the era of my most severe attacks, and shortly before I entered menopause, a gynecologist decided that my headache symptoms might well be linked to a hormone deficiency. He started me on a traditional regimen of cyclical oral hormone supplements (made up of the lowest possible conjugated estrogen [Premarin] dose for three weeks, to be followed by a one-week course of progesterone [Provera]). At the time, I knew very little about the migraine–hormone connection, but my general reading led me to believe this doctor might be setting me on a risky course. Desperate for any relief, however, I decided to follow his advice. When I began the hormone supplements, I was taking no other medication except occasional over-the-counter antihistamine. After trying this hormone regimen for only about one and a half cycles, I decided that the severe nausea I was experiencing every evening was too high a price to pay for an ill-conceived experiment. I had noticed no change in my migraine symptoms, which continued to be quite debilitating.

Not until several years later, after I had informed myself thoroughly about the migraine–hormone link, did I try hormone supplements again. In the interim, I had started taking the antidepressant Prozac and had shed most of my severe attacks. Even with the Prozac, however, I had to remain on a very restrictive diet to avoid symptoms and noticed that I continued to experience an especially vulnerable phase—a few days every four or five weeks during which the consumption of any offending foods might still trigger very debilitating symptoms. This vulnerable phase continued even after I ceased having menstrual periods. My headache diary finally allowed me to realize that these remaining attacks occurred at the same time as other "premenstrual" symptoms, presumably when my natural estrogen level took a dive.

The next time I tried hormone supplements, under the direction of my family practitioner, I started just one hormone at a time—first an estrogen patch (.05 mg estradiol), followed by oral testosterone, and lastly oral progesterone—until finally, after several months, I was taking all three hormones together. Even with an estrogen patch that delivers a continuous low-dose of a different form of that hormone, I found that the evening nausea returned when I changed the patch as often as usually is recommended.*

With my doctor's approval, I have worked out my own schedule, changing the patch every four to five days (instead of the three-to-four-day interval recommended by the manufacturer) as I take into account my body's own natural supply of the hormone at the time. This seems to be a good schedule for me, judging from the fact that I have lost both my hot flashes and my last remaining troublesome migraines—the ones that kept appearing every four to five weeks, seemingly when my natural estrogen level fell. After that loss I felt brave enough to cut my Prozac dose back from two-thirds to one-half capsule. (Other female sufferers may be interested in knowing that estrogen supplements often intensify the effects of antidepressants, sometimes calling for a dosage reduction.) Adding the progesterone didn't seem to affect my headache symptoms one way or the other.

I asked my doctor to add testosterone to my hormone regimen, and I happily report that my remaining headache symptoms have lessened significantly as a result. My daily testosterone dose is ten milligrams, in accordance with my doctor's recommendations, although because of my own caution I started at five milligrams every other day and gradually worked up from there. After more than two years on this regimen, I'm noticing no unpleasant side effects.

The only really troublesome downside to my current hormone replacement therapy is a somewhat greater tendency toward low blood sugar than before—not surprising, considering that both Prozac and estrogen are known to affect the way the body uses sugar. As long as I am very careful to avoid getting really hungry, I feel very well these days.

The Big Picture: *Variations on a Lemonade Recipe*

In summary, keep the following points in mind when you are trying to relieve hormone-related headache symptoms:

1. Use a headache diary to pinpoint the vulnerable phase of your cycle.
2. Take extra precautions to avoid triggers during this time each month.

*Eventually I discovered that daily low-dose aspirin therapy relieved most of my estrogen-associated migraine symptoms. Chapter 10 gives more detailed information on this therapy.

3. For premenstrual or menstrual headaches consider using—
   a. NSAIDs or cyproheptadine (Periactin) on a regular basis, as needed—usually four to seven days a month; and/or one of the popular preventive medications discussed in Chapter 10, either on a daily basis or simply during your most vulnerable phase.
   b. Hormone supplements (estrogen alone or with progesterone and/or testosterone) during this susceptible phase, or testosterone alone on a continuous basis.
   c. In stubborn cases, one of the stronger preventives discussed on pages 110,111.
4. For symptoms related to the pill consider—
   a. Using a lower-dose estrogen preparation or a progesterone-only formulation.
   b. Switching to a different type of contraception.
5. For posthysterectomy or menopausal migraine in which symptoms start or worsen after beginning hormone replacement therapy, consider—
   a. Lowering your estrogen dose and switching to a continuous rather than cyclical schedule.
   b. Switching from conjugated estrogen to a synthetic form of the hormone.
   c. Changing from oral estrogen to the skin patch.
   d. Adding testosterone to your regimen.
   e. Adding low-dose aspirin therapy.
6. For menopausal headaches in those not using hormone supplements, consider—
   a. Starting continuous, low-dose estrogen therapy, especially if you notice signs of a deficiency or if your worst attacks seem to occur about the time you experience symptoms that remind you of premenstrual syndrome.
   b. Instead of, or in addition to, estrogen, beginning testosterone supplementation, particularly if you are experiencing deficiency symptoms.
7. Make only one change per cycle so that the effect of each can be experienced and judged on its own merits (in case you and your doctor decide to implement any of these suggestions).

Balance to Be Achieved

To reach the proper hormone levels for your particular stage in life so that headache symptoms and other signs of hormone dysfunction are relieved.

Chapter 8

Disorders That Muddy the Water

Mimicry, Masquerade, and Mutual Interaction

Reasons for Misdiagnosis

Because there are no definitive tests to "prove" the presence of migraine, its diagnosis remains one of exclusion (as Chapter 1 explains). In addition, a wide array of possible symptoms can, and often does, accompany the primary symptom of headache—symptoms that vary tremendously from one sufferer to another, and frequently even from one attack to another in the same sufferer. To further complicate the situation, many of the symptoms of migraine occur in various other disorders as well. For all of these reasons—plus others that were considered in Chapter 1 (including poor communication skills on the part of physicians and their failure to keep abreast of the latest medical research)—there is an extraordinary possibility for misdiagnosis when dealing with migraine, resulting in many legitimate cases of migraine being mistaken for other conditions and vice versa.

This chapter looks at some of the most common, as well as some of the most complex, instances in which this diagnostic confusion concerning migraine takes place.

Migraine Accompaniments and Equivalents

One primary reason for the complications in migraine diagnosis is that the illness takes so many different forms. If you have compared notes with other sufferers, you are probably aware that the headache itself not only can vary in location and severity, but that it can also be accompanied by a whole set of diverse and sometimes bizarre symptoms in many other parts of the body. These nonheadache symptoms often are every bit as painful as, and even more frightening than, the headache. (For that reason, I personally object to the term "migraine headache," preferring the more inclusive and realistic term "migraine attack.")

115

When these nonheadache symptoms occur as part of a full-blown attack, they are called "accompaniments." When they show up without the headache, as happens fairly often both in sufferers who have endured full-blown attacks in the past, as well as in first-timers, they are called "equivalents." The appearance of these out-of-context symptoms may puzzle both doctor and patient, neither of whom is thinking in terms of a headache-free migraine attack.

Types of Accompaniments/Equivalents

Let's consider briefly the main forms that these symptoms may take. Experts sometimes divide them into the following three classes:

1. *Neurological*—These include several types of symptoms: sensory problems, such as the familiar visual distortions (narrowing field of vision, bright lights), numbness, and disturbed hearing or taste; motor problems, such as dizziness and poor balance; and also disorders of higher function, such as confusion or amnesia.
2. *Visceral*—Abdominal pain, sometimes quite severe and accompanied by chills and sweating, or by nausea and/or diarrhea, is the most common of this type; irregular heart beat and transient chest pain also may occur.
3. *Perceptual*—Sometimes called "Alice in Wonderland Syndrome," this class includes such bizarre symptoms as seeing distorted shapes or sizes, objects with parts missing, or stationary objects that seem to be moving.

Identifying and Dealing with Equivalents

When any of these symptoms appears without headache, a migraine diagnosis definitely should be considered, especially if there is a personal or family history of the disorder. Besides a positive history, another strong clue to the presence of such equivalents is an association of symptoms with exposure to traditional migraine triggers—such things as eating chocolate, drinking alcohol, taking an airplane trip, or having a tooth filled. Of course, such an association usually can be made only by an alert sufferer and only after repeated episodes.

Abdominal migraine, one of the visceral equivalents listed above, is now recognized as a rare occurrence in children, but its appearance among adults is even less frequent. More commonly sufferers of this childhood malady grow up to see their abdominal symptoms change into the traditional headache-based form of migraine. A more common childhood equivalent is thought to be motion sickness; this condition, too, often evolves into a more traditional form of the disorder as the sufferer ages.

Visual migraine (an experience of the aura but without a headache following) probably is the most common equivalent in adults. It frequently
occurs in those middle-aged or older, some, but not all, of whom had full-
blown migraine attacks earlier in life. In about 15% of those who suffer
from visual migraine, symptoms may appear suddenly as if out of the blue;
more often though, they build gradually. Numbness, another common
migraine equivalent, likewise can appear suddenly, but more commonly it
spreads gradually, perhaps from cheeks to lips to tongue, for instance, and
then may "march" to another area of the body. These entire equivalency
attacks may last anywhere from 15 minutes to several hours.

With our current lack of specific diagnostic tests for migraine, regrettably
the only way to zero in on these migraine equivalents is by investigating and
ruling out other disorders with similar symptoms. In the case of abdominal
migraine, for example, depending on the specific symptoms, a doctor might
want to do a workup for appendicitis, gallbladder disease, or irritable bowel
syndrome before feeling sufficiently confident to make a diagnosis. Such an
approach obviously can be frustrating and expensive for the patient, but it is
the best one we have right now. A doctor who really listens to a patient's
symptoms and takes a thorough history probably will pick up some helpful
clues that will allow him to keep testing at a minimum.

Individual Equivalency Experiences

Now that the worst of my migraine symptoms have been eliminated
through a combination of dietary changes, Prozac, and hormone supplements, I continue to experience occasional episodes of unexplained fatigue
and mild nausea. These usually occur during the late afternoon and evening
of the day following some dietary indiscretion. Because of the timing of
these spells following dietary provocations, I assume them to be migraine
equivalents, the relatively mild remnants of my formerly debilitating attacks.
One of my female friends tells me that she has similar episodes. She is a
lifelong migraineur who has noted the gradual disappearance of her severe
attacks as she approached midlife. Even when she was experiencing severe
attacks at a younger age, however, these spells of fatigue and nausea sometimes occurred—almost always in the evening as indeed they do now.

Dr. Charles Aring, a migraineur and retired physician from the University of Cincinnati School of Medicine, describes the way his migraine symptoms have changed over the course of his life. In a recent article, he confirms
what many migraineurs have observed—that symptoms often take different
forms during the various stages of one's life. Now in his 80s, Dr. Aring has
episodes consisting of a visual aura accompanied by impaired thinking and
speaking, but often without the headache he had in earlier years. This

knowedgeable patient understands the nature of his symptoms and seems to take them in stride, but such equivalency experiences often cause confusion and concern, especially in older individuals who might not ever have experienced full-blown attacks.

Mistaken for Migraine

The following illnesses have symptoms so similar to some of the characteristics of migraine that sufferers and/or their doctors may confuse the two.

Allergy

The exact relationship between allergy and migraine continues to puzzle experts, and, clearly, agreement on the subject is lacking. Certainly not all allergy sufferers have migraine, just as the reverse is true. In fact, the migraine prone seem to have no more allergy symptoms than the general population, but in those who do suffer from allergies, even a relatively mild allergic reaction can trigger a migraine attack. Even though no one understands exactly how and why this interaction takes place, it occurs frequently enough to suggest that any migraineur who believes she has allergy triggers would be wise to seek treatment to bring allergic symptoms under reasonable control. Such treatment may require allergy testing followed by desensitization shots, or merely the avoidance of allergens while taking antihistamines or a newer medication called cromolyn sodium. Any of these treatments that your physician might recommend would be appropriate for you as a migraineur.

There is, however, one medication sometimes used in allergy treatment that is not wise for use by migraineurs. Decongestants, often recommended to relieve allergic congestion, are also known to constrict blood vessels and to stimulate the central nervous system, and should therefore probably be avoided by migraineurs. Another point to keep in mind is that allergy tests (whether blood, scratch, or interdermal) should not be performed either during or shortly after a migraine attack. It is best to wait a few days to allow elevated histamine levels to return to normal in order to avoid skewing test results.

And what about "allergy headaches"? Although many of us believe that we suffer from these, experts disagree about whether or not such an animal even exists. Many migraine symptoms—including runny or stuffy nose, watery eyes, temporary hearing loss, or facial pain that seems to be coming from the sinus cavities—mimic allergic reactions and can confuse diagnosis. One primary difference is that these symptoms when caused by allergies tend to occur soon after exposure to the offending substance, whereas the same symptoms when associated with migraine are more likely to be delayed.

The migraine literature suggests that most sufferers do not improve after receiving treatment for their allergies. My husband certainly seems to be an exception to this rule. His headaches, most of which seem to be triggered by exposure to either airborne or dietary mold, improved dramatically after he had skin tests followed by a two-year series of desensitivization injections.

Sinus Infection

This condition, actually a bacterial infection, does sometimes result in headache symptoms. Such sinus headaches are rare, however, and are usually accompanied by a fever and persistent facial pain. Sometimes, thick, colored nasal mucous is present. Evidently some doctors tend to confuse this condition with migraine. Severe facial pain can be predominant in either condition, but it behaves differently in each.

In sinus headache, the pain tends to continue until the blockage is cleared and may remain relatively constant for as long as several weeks. A CT scan of the sinus cavities often will identify any existing problems. A new incisionless surgical procedure can easily help to pinpoint the causes for some previously mysterious cases of sinus pain, according to Dr. William Keane of Philadelphia's Thomas Jefferson University. Keane points out that an endoscope inserted in either nostril can be used to diagnose and treat sinus problems, finding obstructions in nasal passages not identified by previous methods.

In migraine, the pain builds more gradually, peaks, and then typically clears up within a few hours to a few days. Usual treatments for sinus infection include decongestants and antibiotics, neither of which is called for in combating migraine.

Cervicogenic Headache

This type of headache, which is caused by a structural abnormality, such as herniated disk or a bone spur that presses on a nerve in the neck or back, is frequently confused with common migraine. If one investigates closely, however, there are some differences between the two disorders, allowing for correct diagnosis and treatment. Pain and/or numbness in the neck, shoulders, and/or arms is much more prominent in cervicogenic headache than in common migraine. Frequently this pain is accompanied by some restriction of movement in the neck. Although neck and back pain and stiffness may appear in migraineurs during attacks, these symptoms almost always disappear between episodes.

Cervicogenic pain tends to start in the back of the head (although it may spread elsewhere), whereas the pain of common migraine typically begins in or near the eyes. Furthermore, when the former type of headache is one-sided, it tends to remain on the same side, whereas the pain of one-sided migraine may alternate from side to side, or spread from one side to both. Common migraine is much more likely to run in families than is this other type of headache, and both photophobia (light sensitivity) and vomiting tend to be more severe in migraine.

If symptoms indicate the likelihood of cervicogenic headache, a neurologist can usually establish a definite diagnosis by means of a scan (CT or MRI) of the neck and/or back. Some of the supposed migraine thought to respond to physical therapy or chiropractic treatment may in fact constitute this other disorder.

Please be aware of the possibility that one individual could suffer from *both* of these types of headache. Thus, even if you have a family or personal history of migraine, you might want to consider an examination for cervicogenic headache if you begin to experience pain, numbness, or restricted movement in your neck and/or arms between migraine attacks or if these symptoms become part of your attacks for the first time.

Inner-Ear Disorders

Two disorders that closely resemble migraine are the inner ear conditions of vertigo and Meniere's Syndrome. Both of these afflictions involve dizziness or lightheadedness combined with balance problems or unsteady gait. Meniere's also includes ringing or other ear noises (called tinnitus) in one or both ears, temporary hearing loss that sometimes becomes permanent, nausea and vomiting, headache, and sometimes fainting. It should come as no great surprise that these symptoms sound more than slightly familiar. Many migraineurs experience vertigo, commonly during attacks, but occasionally between them as well. Symptoms of Meniere's are exactly the same as those of a severe form of migraine that is called "basilar artery migraine," because at one time it was thought to originate near an artery by that name. Experts observe that these inner-ear disorders respond quite well to the same medications that are used to treat migraine, and indeed some are beginning to wonder whether or not these so-called ear conditions are not simply migraine variants or equivalents.

At the very least, migraine and inner-ear disorders are very closely related. In addition to having similar symptoms, both tend to occur periodically, are often on one side of the head, and are experienced predominantly by women. Both appear to involve blood vessel instability, but may well be primarily neurotransmitter disorders.

When an ear specialist originally misdiagnosed my condition as Meniere's Syndrome, I was surprised to get partial but immediate relief from the antihistamine he gave me to dry up the fluid in my inner ear, a process that I had been told would take from weeks to months. It was in that serendipitous fashion that I discovered the value of garden-variety antihistamines in migraine treatment, a discovery that didn't fully sink in until much later.

Retinal Detachment

This very serious eye problem can closely resemble a visual aura or so-called ocular migraine (aura *without* the headache). Both may include seeing bright flashes of light and either blurred vision or the loss of a portion of the visual field. Neither involves eye pain. One distinction is that in the case of a detached retina, floaters—light or dark specks, spots, or lines that appear to move around—are often present. People who have had cataract surgery are at an increased risk of developing this condition. It is always considered a medical emergency, and those who suspect they are experiencing it should report to an ophthalmologist or an emergency room immediately.

Meningitis

This condition is caused by either a viral or bacterial infection in the membrane that surrounds the brain and spinal cord. It can be relatively mild and may even clear up without treatment; on the other hand this infection sometimes is life threatening, requiring immediate and intensive treatment. Meningitis often occurs as a complication of an infection present elsewhere in the body, such as in the ears, sinuses, or even a tooth. Both diabetes and alcoholism predispose a person to this disorder, as does any disease that significantly weakens the immune system (AIDS, for example). Symptoms of meningitis can be very similar to some of those in migraine—including severe headache, vomiting, light sensitivity, confusion, drowsiness, and possibly a stiff neck. But with meningitis (unlike migraine), at least some of the symptoms come on rather suddenly, and fever is always present. In the bacterial variety, blood tests will show an increased white cell count. Often a lumbar puncture (spinal tap) is needed to establish a specific diagnosis.

Encephalitis

Presenting another emergency medical situation, this condition stems from an infection of the nerve cells of the brain itself. An infected mosquito or tick can be responsible for spreading the disease. Symptoms are similar to meningitis, and indeed the two can occur together or at least within a short time of each another as the internal infection spreads. Fever and sudden onset are the primary symptoms differentiating this disorder from migraine. Again, blood tests and a spinal tap are called for if encephalitis is suspected.

Reyes Syndrome

This disorder primarily strikes children between the ages of two and 18, usually following within a week of the onset of a viral infection such as a cold, influenza, or chicken pox. Symptoms from the initial illness may begin to improve before the appearance of persistent nausea, vomiting, and gradually worsening confusion. Although individual symptoms may resemble migraine, the pattern in which they appear is quite different.

Because medical experts believe that aspirin may lead to this condition, they advise against its use for treating viral infections in youngsters under 18. In fact, aspirin should be avoided in treating all headache in this age group, since the exact cause of the symptoms will be difficult, if not impossible, to pinpoint. The NSAIDs appear safe.

Multiple Sclerosis

This nerve fiber disease that commonly strikes young people between 20 and 40 can begin with migraine-like symptoms, including coordination and balance problems, pain and tingling in various parts of the body (including headache or other facial pain), blurred or double vision, fatigue, and mental confusion. As in migraine, symptoms can come and go in an episodic fashion, and there may be long periods of remission between spells. Keys to detection are a family history of the disease and the fact that heat, such as a hot bath or strenuous activity on a hot day, severely worsens symptoms. An MRI scan is helpful in establishing this diagnosis.

Stroke

Both migraine and stroke seem to involve increased platelet aggregation, the tendency of blood platelets to clump together too readily, and migraine symptoms often bear a striking similarity to those of stroke. This is particularly true when the perceptual or mental distortions described under equivalencies are present. Since migraine attacks are episodic and tend to recur over time in the same individuals, the periodic reappearance of the same symptoms without lingering disability between attacks is one hallmark of that disorder. But in an initial attack, particularly one appearing in a person over 40, differentiating between migraine and stroke sometimes can be rather tricky. When neurological migraine equivalents (no headache) appear for the first time in an older individual, many physicians believe the situation calls for a complete neurological examination to rule out the presence of stroke, which is more common in that age group than among the younger population.

Even though in some cases the symptoms of migraine and stroke are very similar, there are usually some hints in the way these symptoms appear that help us to differentiate between the two conditions. Dr. C. M. Fisher, neurologist at Massachusetts General Hospital, studied 120 patients who had rather mysterious spells—neurological symptoms in the face of normal cerebral angiograms (brain X-rays). Only half of those studied also had headache. Dr. Fisher, now considered an authority in differentiating between migraine and stroke, emphasizes the following distinctions between the two conditions: In stroke or mini-stroke (the latter technically is called TIA, short for transient ischemic attack), symptoms typically appear suddenly in full-blown form, whereas in migraine symptoms usually come on more gradually. Migraine symptoms are said to "build"; for example, the field of vision is likely to narrow gradually, or numbness may progress or "march" from one area to another over the course of about 15–30 minutes. The most confusing patients—about one-fourth of migraine sufferers— experience a sudden onset of symptoms exactly like those of stroke or TIA. In such patients, complete neurological workups, including angiograms, scans, and blood work, may well be necessary to differentiate between the two conditions.

In migraineurs, these neurological symptoms typically disappear between attacks without treatment. When neurological deficits (such as narrowed field of vision or hearing loss, for example) remain indefinitely, as they do in some sufferers in spite of normal test results, the symptoms often can be relieved by means of anticoagulant drugs—that is, with drugs that decrease the clumping tendency of platelets. Low doses of aspirin or a drug called dipyridamole (sold as Pyridamole, Persantine, or as a generic) are often recommended for these patients, as well as in sufferers who have frequent attacks with neurological symptoms. Low-dose aspirin therapy decreased the frequency of migraine attacks by 20% in an impressively large and well controlled study of male migraineurs who were followed over a five-year period; the aspirin treatment significantly cut stroke risk in this group as well. Some specialists prefer a combination of low-dose aspirin therapy and the calcium blocker verapamil (Calan) in these groups.

In the younger population, stroke is a very rare occurrence, but some studies show that about one-fourth of people under 40 who do have strokes are migraineurs—a much greater association than can be explained by chance. A group of Danish neurologists recently studied stroke risk in young migraineurs over a ten-year period. These doctors recommend that young sufferers, especially males, who experience neurological symptoms and who have known cardiovascular risk factors, such as obesity, high cholesterol levels, and/or high blood pressure, or are smokers, should have a complete medical workup for stroke.

Experts don't yet understand the exact relationship between these two conditions, but it has long been suspected that migraineurs, especially those with obvious neurological symptoms, have a higher than average risk of stroke. Findings released by the Physicians' Health Study in late 1991 confirm that male migraineurs (unfortunately only male subjects were included in the study) have double the risk of stroke found in the general population. (Not to panic, for even with double the risk, the odds of actually suffering a stroke are still small, especially in the absence of other risk factors.)

In light of these recent research findings linking migraine and stroke, common sense tells us that as migraineurs we should take risk factors seriously and adjust our lifestyles accordingly. Of course, if we heed the warnings, we are likely to receive positive reinforcement for our efforts because the very same lifestyle changes that will reduce our long-term stroke risk should bring about a more immediate improvement in our migraine symptoms. Surely that's a win–win situation if ever there was one!

Epilepsy

For decades, medical scientists have suspected that migraine and epilepsy share a similar cause, probably a malfunction in the cortex (the outer layer of the cerebrum, which is rich in nerve cells). Even with sophisticated modern diagnostic instruments, however, there still is no real understanding about what that common factor might be. It is clear, however, that there sometimes is an overlap between symptoms of the two conditions, making diagnosis difficult, especially in children. These common symptoms include visual distortions, balance disturbances, and numbness, among others. The presence of actual seizures definitively points to epilepsy, but a fair number of patients have both migraine and full-blown epilepsy with seizures, an association that many believe occurs too often to be a mere coincidence. The two conditions sometimes respond favorably to the same medications.

Brain Tumor

This disorder no doubt is the one most feared by migraineurs, especially before the cause of sometimes quite bizarre symptoms is diagnosed. Yet, experts tell us, headache is seldom an early symptom of a brain tumor—a condition usually first signaled by seizures, confusion, or fainting. Most agree that fewer than 1% of patients who come to a physician complaining of severe headache are found to have a tumor. In the presence of such a growth, head pain is usually localized, and often weakness on one side of the body is apparent during examination. Of course, if a tumor is even suspected, CT or MRI (popular abbreviations for computerized axial tomography and magnetic resonance imaging) scans will be ordered, since they are the best methods for detecting such a condition.

Bleeding Aneurysm

This is another rare but potentially fatal headache condition that could possibly be confused with migraine. There are some major differences, however. Usually symptoms from this disorder begin suddenly, often during exertion (as in fact do a small number of migraines), but with an aneurysm there is nearly always some mental confusion or disorientation. This condition nearly always occurs in someone over 35 years of age. If there is any question about a diagnosis, a scan and lumbar puncture probably should be done, since these symptoms can warn of a future rupture.

Multiple Chemical Sensitivity

This disorder shares some similarity with migraine, including symptoms of dizziness, headache, rapid heartbeat, inability to concentrate, and hypersensitivity to chemicals/odors among others. (Refer to Chapter 4 for a brief discussion of this illness and its possible relationship to migraine.)

Complicating Disorders

The following conditions, although not actually mistaken for migraine, do interact with the headache disorder in some rather significant ways and so should be of special interest to sufferers.

Depression and Anxiety

Research studies link migraine to both depression and anxiety, but here again there is a lack of understanding about the relationship among these three conditions; estimates of the exact extent of the association vary. We do have evidence, however, that migraine sufferers experience both of these mood disorders to a significantly greater degree than the general population. The best estimates are that between 20 and 40% of migraineurs also suffer from depression, compared with between three and six percent of the general population.

In one large study, psychiatrists at Yale University followed 47 male and 47 female subjects for eight years (while the subjects were in their twenties). Of the 61 migraineurs in the group, 20% also had a history of both anxiety and depression, but only 6% of the nonmigraineurs suffered from those mood disturbances.

Research shows, as well, that the signs of anxiety and depression (these two often appear together resulting in what is described as a kind of "anxious depression") frequently occur even before or shortly after headache symptoms appear, ruling out the possibility, at least in most cases, that the headache disorder causes the mood symptoms. Of course, struggling with chronic migraine *is* a stressful experience that indeed can worsen depressive symptoms. The type of depression that occurs most often among migraineurs, however, seems to be biologically determined and inherited rather than strictly a response to life stressors. It may be that the biological factors that predispose a person to depression also predispose to migraine. (Some experts speculate that depression is more likely to accompany common migraine [migraine without aura] than classic migraine, although the validity of this theory seems questionable in light of current thinking about the apparent overlap between these types of headache.)

It only makes sense that this high rate of depression among migraineurs should be a major consideration in selecting a preventive medication. However, depressive symptoms frequently are not obvious in migraine sufferers, especially in the context of a superficial meeting—a fact that may complicate the job of identifying the best treatment. The association between these two disorders is so strong, however, that some experts recommend routinely taking a detailed psychiatric history to avoid overlooking depressive symptoms. If low level depression or anxiety have been present since youth, even the migraineur herself may not be aware that her mood is anything but normal. (*See* Chapter 11 for a further discussion of this topic.)

Thyroid Disorders

Thyroid hormones are known to interact with serotonin and noradrenalin, two of the brain chemicals implicated in migraine. Patients with hyperthyroidism (the condition in which too much thyroid hormone is produced) show an increased sensitivity to tyramine, a recognized trigger of dietary migraine. Thus this condition can act as a threshold-lowering agent for those predisposed to migraine. For these reasons, a complete thyroid profile (via a simple blood test) should be included as part of the physical exam done to evaluate a beginning or worsening migraine condition. Patients who take thyroid supplements to correct an underactive thyroid should be sure to have blood hormone levels checked at least yearly, or sooner if migraine symptoms appear to be worsening.

Fever

In some sufferers, a fever associated with any illness may trigger a migraine attack. (Indeed, in some sensitive people even a minor infection occurring without a fever can be enough to cause a headache.) This happenstance, when one disorder superimposes itself on another, can create a confusing scenario, especially when it occurs in children. If you're an adult migraineur who reacts in this manner, however, you will soon catch on to what's happening. A special caution is in order when treating such attacks because vasoconstrictive medications often used as abortives can be dangerous if used in the presence of fever; be sure to get your doctor's okay before using ergot, ergot derivatives (such as Cafergot or DHE), or even Midrin under these circumstances.

Blood Sugar Disorders

Strong evidence links fluctuating blood sugar levels with the occurrence of migraines. In evaluating sufferers whose headaches went into remission, British expert Dr. J. N. Blau tentatively connects this loss in some subjects to their development or treatment of diabetes, a condition involving overly *high* blood sugar levels. Others have long observed that falling blood sugar levels seem to be a specific trigger for some migraineurs and a threshold-lowering factor for many others.

Technically speaking, only about 5% of the population suffer from hypoglycemia (low blood sugar, a disorder in which sugar levels fall below 40 mg per deciliter of blood), but many experts believe that falling blood sugar levels can set off migraine attacks in susceptible people even if that "magic" number is not reached, and studies clearly show that long periods of fasting often do trigger attacks. Anecdotal evidence strongly suggests that inadequate meals may lead to symptoms as well.

You might suspect that you have a tendency toward this disorder if you frequently experience one or more of the following symptoms shortly before mealtimes or when meals have been delayed or missed: unusual weakness or fatigue, irritability or nervousness, trembling, dizziness, excessive sweating, mild confusion, or palpitations. (To review tips for avoiding attacks triggered by low blood sugar, reread Chapter 4.)

Certain medications can cause or worsen hypoglycemia. Antidepressants used as migraine preventives can have this effect, as can estrogen supplements and oral contraceptives. If you suspect that a medication you are taking is causing this problem, and if you are unable to live with it comfortably after implementing the dietary suggestions in Chapter 4, you may want to check with your doctor about a possible alternative.

Platelet Hyperaggregation

Many experts believe that this condition—simply the medical name for blood platelets that clump together too readily—is a threshold-lowering factor for migraine. (The speculation is that when platelets clump together, they "dump" their serotonin content, thus setting off the migraine reaction.) This theory was supported by results of the previously mentioned Physicians' Health Study showing that male migraineurs who took an aspirin a day achieved a 20% reduction in their migraine frequency. Other research demonstrates that far lower aspirin doses can achieve the same benefit with less risk. (The drug is a potent gastrointestinal irritant, and larger doses, taken regularly, seem to *interefere* with the body's own natural pain fighting substance, thus worsening migraine.)

Preliminary trials suggest that Vitamin-E supplementation may well have a similar anticlumping effect. Regular aerobic exercise and a low-fat diet also seem to result in healthier platelet behavior. Smoking, on the other hand, is known to cause increased platelet stickiness.

Iron Deficiency Anemia

This disorder may contribute to dietary migraine by causing a deficiency in monoamine oxidase (MAO), the enzyme that seems to play an important role in breaking down vasoactive substances in foods. Some research on the enzyme suggests that iron supplements given to correct anemia increase body levels of MAO even when they don't succeed in raising blood hemoglobin. Check with your doctor before taking iron supplements, however, since too much iron can be harmful, and the supplements often act as gastric irritants. Dietary iron is better absorbed when Vitamin C-rich foods are eaten at the same time, but arranging this combination may pose somewhat of a challenge for the severe migraineur, who probably will not be able to tolerate citrus. Certain raw vegetables, such as carrots and green peppers, and almost any raw fruit can help to boost natural Vitamin C levels and thus aid iron absorption.

The Big Picture: *Migraine and Other Disorders*

In summary, differentiating between migraine and other medical conditions demands knowledge, patience, and skill because migraine symptoms are quite varied and resemble the symptoms of many other illnesses. Doctors who are unaware that the headache of migraine usually is not preceded by a specific aura and that it sometimes is two-sided are most likely to make an incorrect diagnosis. Migraine is especially misleading to both sufferer and physician when its nonheadache symptoms occur without the usual headache. Sometimes lab tests and/or scans are necessary to make a diagnosis, but a good doctor can learn a great deal about your illness by carefully listening to you and performing a thorough manual examination in the office.

Some common physical and emotional conditions can interact with and complicate migraine. If you have symptoms of thyroid imbalance, depression and/or anxiety, blood sugar disorders, iron deficiency anemia, or platelet hyperaggregation, then it is important to the long-term management of your migraine condition that these symptoms be carefully evaluated and treated.

Balance to Be Achieved

To obtain an accurate diagnosis of migraine and other conditions that have similar symptoms without undergoing unnecessary medical tests; and to receive proper diagnosis and treatment for other conditions that may worsen migraine.

Chapter 9

Nonheadache Drugs Cause Trouble

Is Anybody Checking?

The Thigh Bone's Connected to . . . Who Knows What

We migraineurs seeking medical treatment to relieve symptoms of other conditions quite naturally tend to be somewhat single minded, perhaps forgetting for a time about our headache disorder as we concentrate on our aching knee, or whatever. If you remember the discussion of Blau's study on "losing migraine" from Chapter 3, perhaps you recall that some of the migraineurs interviewed traced the disappearance of their headache symptoms to the time they started taking medication for other conditions. Chapter 10 on medical treatments mentions the accidental discovery that certain medications developed to treat heart and blood pressure problems also bring significant relief to migraine symptoms.

Indeed, we have learned that this unintended action between nonheadache medications and headache can work both ways—either to relieve or worsen symptoms. This two-way process is extremely complex and frequently takes an unexpected turn or two—something that really shouldn't surprise us considering that migraine seems to have its origins in the brain, the organ that acts as the command and control center for our entire body, or, as Norman Cousins describes it in *Head First*, as our "master apothecary."

Many migraine experts name nonheadache medications as threshold-setters for migraine, that is, as significant determinants of the individual sufferer's vulnerability to attacks. Thus it came as a major surprise and disappointment to me to discover that very little comprehensive research and writing has been done on this important link. The one bright spot in this otherwise black hole of medical literature is an article by Dr. Glen D. Solomon, entitled "Concomitant Medical Disease and Headache," which appears in the May, 1991, edition of *The Medical Clinics of North America* (Vol. 75, No. 3). You can find this publication in a medical library or order it through the interlibrary loan system. Dr. Solomon's article is certainly well worth reading for anyone who is receiving medical treatment for one or more ongoing conditions in addition to migraine. In writing this chapter, I am heavily indebted to Dr. Solomon because, except for his article, references to this significant link are sparse indeed.

Whose Responsibility Is It Anyway?

In view of this near dearth of information, it may be somewhat naive of us to expect our doctors to be well versed on this important link between migraine and nonheadache medications. We would like to believe that we could always count on them to look after our welfare in a comprehensive way, juggling knowledge of our various illnesses with the side effects of all our medications to assure the best possible interaction among them. Unfortunately, at least in this particular case, such complete reliance on the medical profession just won't work.

It becomes our job as patients, then, to keep tabs on our overall response to medication, being mindful whether our headache symptoms change, either for good or ill, as a result of medications we are taking for other conditions or, indeed, whether our headache medicines tend to aggravate other medical disorders. An equally important part of that responsibility consists of making our doctors aware of any changes that we notice. After all, in their defense, let's remember that neither are they with us 24 hours a day, nor are they able to read our minds. Sometimes we act as if both were the case!

An Advocate's Dilemma

Medical literature recognizes that various medications taken for many different conditions can either cause or worsen headache symptoms in susceptible people. *The Physicians' Desk Reference* (PDR) lists headache as a possible side effect of numerous medications, but because that manual does not usually specify the type of headache that may result, it is difficult to predict the effect that migraineurs will experience from some of these drugs. Little controlled research has been conducted to show specifically which drugs actually may cause or worsen migraine. Therefore we are left, at least in many cases, to rely on theory and anecdotal reports (what patients say about their reactions) in judging which drugs may be risky for us.

Considering this lack of hard evidence, someone writing about migraine finds herself in a disturbing quandary. The traditional medical establishment chooses to remain silent about possible drug reactions not firmly established by research, but as a migraineur now acting as an advocate for other sufferers, I feel compelled to present probabilities, based on theoretical assumptions, in addition to that data widely accepted by the medical community.

Therefore I am choosing to include as cautionary that class of drugs known as "sympathomimetics"—i.e., adrenaline-producing or -releasing medications—based both on theory and on evidence that patients taking monoamine–oxidase inhibitors react adversely to these drugs. (You may recall from Chapter 2 that these patients, taking a certain type of antidepressant, react badly to many of the same foods that bother dietary migraineurs.) Although these adrenaline-producing or -releasing drugs may not necessarily cause problems for all migraineurs in all instances, the possibility of problems with their use convinces me of the fairness of warning other sufferers of that potential. *So that you will know which drugs are mentioned on this somewhat controversial basis, they will be marked with an asterisk.* Other drugs labeled as risky have either been so shown by research and/or are widely accepted as risky by many migraine authorities.

Pharmaceutical Troublemakers

At least in theory, drugs can act in several ways to complicate the migraine scenario. Since migraine is thought to involve an overly sensitive central nervous system as well as a poorly regulated vascular network, migraineurs should approach with extreme caution any medication that further stimulates either of these systems. Other likely sources of trouble are drugs that lower blood sugar and drugs that increase platelet stickiness or aggregation, as well as drugs that decrease the relative serotonin level in the brain either directly or indirectly, by increasing the level of other brain chemicals and thus changing the delicate balance among them.

If your doctor suggests that you use a drug that acts in any of these ways, you may want to consider asking him for an alternative treatment. Certainly, if headache symptoms either begin or worsen while you are using such a drug, or, indeed, after you begin any new medication, you will want to inform and question your doctor. As Chapter 1 points out, the informed patient is the most likely to receive good medical care, so inform yourself about possible side effects of drugs that you are taking or are considering, but please do not discontinue medications or change the dosage on your own.

Specifically, the following drugs should be approached with caution:

Female Hormones

Headaches frequently worsen in women taking birth control pills or using hormone replacement therapy (HRT) after hysterectomy or menopause. Studies show, in fact, that many women beginning "the pill" soon experience either an initial migraine attack or a worsening of existing symptoms. On the other hand, a smaller number of pill users actually improves while on these very same hormones. Experts usually advise that women whose symptoms worsen while using these hormones should discontinue or alter their use in order to avoid an increased risk of stroke. Some women who cannot tolerate the traditional high-dose estrogen contraceptives avoid symptoms by switching either to a lower-dose estrogen or to a progesterone-only formula, but many will have to use an alternate form of contraception. Specifically, a plunging estrogen level, occurring after previously high levels, seems to be responsible for triggering most pill-related attacks, with headaches commonly occurring on days immediately after estrogen has been stopped. Your gynecologist should be willing to work with you on this, especially if you remind him that you need to avoid rapidly falling estrogen levels; but if he is stymied, then a neurologist with a special interest in migraine should be able to help.

In the case of HRT after menopause or hysterectomy, it again appears that falling estrogen levels are the chief culprit in triggering attacks. Sustained levels that are too high for a particular person can cause problems as well, however. Maintaining relatively even levels of the hormone—levels that are just high enough to control symptoms of hot flashes and fatigue—seems to be the most helpful strategy for avoiding migraine symptoms. Continuous, noncyclical administration is the recommended way to go. The estrogen patch gets the job done nicely and is better tolerated by many women than oral dosing. The accompanying progesterone can be given in one of several different ways, with no apparent effect on migraine symptoms. (For more specific information on the link between female hormones and migraine, *see* Chapter 7.)

Heart and Blood Pressure Remedies

Some of these medications are notorious for causing headaches. Troublemakers include vasodilators, such as nitroglycerine, given for angina (insufficient blood supply to the heart), certain calcium channel blockers, given to correct irregular heart rhythms and/or to lower blood pressure, and the vasodilator antihypertensives hydralazine (sold as Apresazide and other brand names), methyldopa (sold as Aldoclor and Aldoril), and minoxidil (sold as Loniten and Minoxidil), among others. (Rogaine, a dilute form of minoxidil that is applied to the scalp to promote hair growth, does not seem to present a problem for the headache-prone person.) Reserpine, a strong drug usually reserved for unresponsive high blood pressure cases, is known to cause both severe headache and depression. This drug is sold both alone and in numerous combinations under many different brand names. It belongs to a wider family of medications called rauwolfia alkaloid derivatives, all of which are likely to spell trouble for migraineurs.

Among the calcium channel blockers, nifedipine (Adalat or Procardia), nicardipine (Cardene), and nimodipine (Nimotop) have been identified as causing unpleasant daily headaches in some individuals. Nifedipine specifically has been identified as worsening migraine. (Other calcium channel blockers, however, actually seem to be effective migraine preventives.) Diuretics, given to prevent fluid retention and often included in a blood pressure control regimen, have been shown to worsen migraine in rare instances.

Decongestants*

These ingredients that appear in nearly all over-the-counter and prescription cold and sinus preparations—including tablets, capsules, syrups, drops and sprays—stimulate the central nervous system and constrict blood vessels. All such preparations are potentially risky for migraineurs, in spite of the fact that physicians sometimes suggest them for headache symptoms. The PDR lists headache, nausea, and vomiting as possible side effects for most decongestants; for many of these medications, dizziness and palpitations are potential problems as well. In their popular book *Headache Relief,* Drs. Rapoport and Sheftell suggest that decongestants are not appropriate headache medications and may, in fact, make the condition worse because of their effects on blood pressure and circulation.

I personally can testify that migraineurs sometimes experience bizarre and frightening symptoms from using these drugs. Once when using a popular decongestant in the form of a nasal spray, I had repeated episodes of extreme tinnitus (ear noises), reminiscent of battleground noises, that caused me literally to question my sanity. Some sufferers may be able to use these products in moderation without such dramatic ill effects, but caution is definitely in order.

Phenylpropanolamine is the oral decongestant with the greatest effect on blood vessels. This ingredient, often called PPA for short, is contained in Alka-Seltzer Plus, Contac, Dimetapp, Dristan capsules, and many other common cold and sinus preparations. The PDR and other reputable medical

*Labeled as risky for migraineurs on theoretical grounds, not yet supported by research or general concensus.

sources cite severe headache as the most common adverse reaction to PPA. One source describes acute repetitive attacks of severe headaches and vomiting as a result of the use of a nasal decongestant containing this ingredient; the author doesn't call these episodes migraine, but the symptoms of the two certainly are similar.

Another popular oral decongestant is pseudoephedrine, the active ingredient in Sudafed and many similar preparations. Although this particular drug is considered milder and safer than PPA for the average patient, it is still risky for migraineurs because of its vasoconstrictive action.

When headache sufferers need help in dealing with watery secretions caused by allergies or colds, antihistamines are a far safer alternative. However, if you are determined to use a decongestant to combat a stuffy nose, the lesser of the evils may be nose drops, which work largely on a local level, thus minimizing central nervous system absorption. Most nasal sprays and drops, such as Dristan, Sinex, and Neo-Synephrine, rely on phenylephrine hydrochloride as their active ingredient. Longer-lasting products, such as Afrin, Duration, and Neo-Synephrine II, contain a stronger active ingredient and are more likely to cause trouble.

Let's talk possible alternatives. If nasal congestion is a severe but temporary problem (during hay fever season, for instance), you may want to consider using a topical steroid in the form of a prescription nose spray to see you through the crisis. Examples of these relatively new steroid products include flunisolide, sold as Nasalide, and beclomethasone, sold as Vancenase. For a sore throat, regular pain relievers in conjunction with a warm saltwater gargle are probably adequate for most people. For garden-variety coughs, simply doubling up on liquids and using a steam vaporizer should provide some relief. The expectorant ingredient guaifenesin, contained in Hytuss tablets (over-the-counter) or Humibid LA (prescription), is probably safe. For suppressing a cough, the ingredient dextromethorphan, the active ingredient in Hold DM tablets (over-the-counter), may be tolerated by some migraineurs but should be approached cautiously. For bedtime use, in treating a dry (nonproductive) cough, a simple antihistamine tablet might be helpful. As a rule of thumb, antihistamines are safe for migraineurs, but decongestants should be used with great caution, if at all and most cough syrups should be avoided because of their high alcohol content.

Asthma Medication

Adrenaline-producing drugs frequently are used to treat severe asthma attacks. These drugs—such as the old stand-by ephedrine[*] (marketed under such brand names as Bronkotabs, Tedral, and many others) and the newer cousin epinephrine[*] (sold as Bronkaid or Primatene Mist and various other designations)—effectively increase air flow thorough the bronchial tubes. They are available as oral and injectable preparations, as well as bronchodilators, and are used to treat not only asthma, but also chronic bronchitis, emphysema, and other lung diseases. The oral forms of these drugs are even more likely to cause central nervous system symptoms (e.g., headache) than are the aerosols.

Other risky sympathomimetic asthma drugs include albuterol* (Proventil and Ventolin), the similar medicine metaproterenol* (Alupent/Metaprel), as well as isoproterenol* (Isuprel), terbutaline* (Brethine), and isoetharine* (Bronkosol). Potentially troublesome for us is the fact that all of these agents stimulate the sympathetic nervous system, which many think is already overactive in migraineurs. And of further concern, many of these asthma treatments (specifically the bronchodilators and IVs) contain sulfite as a preservative, even though this ingredient has been shown to cause fatal sensitivity reactions, especially among asthmatics, and also to trigger migraine attacks in some people.

It may be best to avoid this class of drugs altogether, perhaps relying instead on intravenous steroids or theophylline to stop a *severe* asthma attack. For ongoing asthma treatment in migraineurs, however, theophylline and other xanthine derivatives, whose chemical composition is very similar to caffeine, are not recommended. Like their caffeine cousin, these xanthines can be useful in the short term, but long-term use appears to worsen migraine. This class of drugs, sold as bronchodilators, oral agents, and enema preparations, is often recommended both to prevent and to interrupt asthma attacks and other bronchial disorders. Theophylline, probably the most popular of these, is sold as a generic or under many different brand names, including Theo-Dur and Theobid.

For ongoing asthma treatment in the headache sufferer, better drugs are now available. Both cromolyn sodium and steroid inhalants are considered safe and effective for asthmatic headache sufferers. Cromolyn sodium (sold as Intal) often is considered the drug of choice for control of mild to moderate asthma symptoms. If a patient's response to this medication is unsatisfactory, then she may be a candidate for a steroid inhalant, a powerful but effective treatment that recent research shows usually does not cause serious side effects, as some might fear. In fact I rush to reassure you: These drugs are *not* closely related to the feared anabolic steroids known to do so much harm to athletes. It is extremely unfortunate that their label confuses and frightens prospective users. These clever aerosol steroids are able to direct their medication right to the lungs and thus largely avoid being

---

*Labeled as risky for migraineurs on theoretical grounds, not yet supported by research or general concensus.

absorbed into the rest of the body. Examples of such products include Beclovent (which contains beclomethasone diproprionate) and Aerobid (whose active ingredient is flunisolide).

If your asthma requires preventive treatment, you might want to consider one of these newer agents, at least on a trial basis, to see whether or not migraine symptoms improve.

Weight-Loss Products

Both prescription and over-the-counter diet aids usually rely on some form of amphetamines to suppress appetite. (People also take these products to combat drowsiness although the PDR specifically warns against this practice.) One of these products, fenfluramine (a prescription drug usually sold under the brand name Pondimin), has been shown in controlled trials to worsen migraine significantly. Since all amphetamines are similar chemically and all act as central nervous system stimulants, probably all should be avoided by cautious migraineurs. Many over-the-counter diet products contain the potent and potentially dangerous central nervous system stimulant phenylpropanolamine (sold as Dexatrim, Dietac, and Appedrine)—the very same PPA discussed under "Decongestants" above.

Other Adrenaline-Producing/Releasing Drugs

The technical, medical name for this class of drugs that either produces adrenaline in the body or causes adrenaline to be released from storage sites is "sympathomimetic." The decongestants, weight-loss products, and airway expanders discussed in this chapter all belong to this large drug category. In addition to the uses already discussed, these adrenaline-producing drugs also are used in treating both the sleep disorder narcolepsy and attention deficit hyperactivity disorder (primarily in children), as well as several different forms of shock.

Specifically, methylphenidate hydrochloride[*] (sold as Ritalin), the amphetamine-like medication frequently used to counteract both hyperactivity and narcolepsy, falls in this general category and is potentially risky for migraineurs. (These conditions often can be helped by antidepressants.) In addition, the drops used to dilate eyes before a vision examination usually contain epinephrine or phenylephrine, adrenaline-releasing drugs with the potential of causing headache. If you must undergo eye dilation, request the weakest effective solution.

---

[*]Labeled as risky for migraineurs on theoretical grounds, not yet supported by research or general concensus.

Some authorities suggest that sensitive individuals who need drugs from this class in emergency situations involving allergic or surgical shock (epinephrine is commonly used), or some other form of physical trauma, such as cardiac arrest, begin with about one-fourth the usual dose. In the case of serious allergic reactions to insect stings, foods, or medications, injected antihistamines often will bring satisfactory relief. Severe migraineurs might be well advised to discuss with their primary-care physicians possible alternatives to these agents in the event of unconsciousness in an emergency scenario. The use of an emergency alert bracelet or necklace to advise minimizing or avoiding this class of drugs might be prudent as well.

General Anesthetics and Other Surgically Related Drugs*

Informal reports from sufferers suggest that migraineurs are especially sensitive to general anesthetics. This is a topic that is difficult to sort out because of the requirement for fasting before receiving such drugs. Only controlled research could establish the cause of the attacks—the fasting or the anesthesia—and apparently this has not been done. (You might want to consider IV feedings before surgery in order to avoid pre- or postsurgical attacks.)

When and if these drugs are needed, some migraine authors believe that minimum doses should be given. At the very least, common sense dictates that orders for abortive migraine medication should be in place beforehand. Better yet, check with the personnel at the nursing station to be sure that the medication is actually available before undergoing the knife or any procedure requiring a general anesthetic. It seems wise to consider other possible drug sensitivities before surgery and to discuss them with your doctor as well. A common precaution is the discontinuation of any "blood thinning" medications well in advance of surgery. These would include the aspirin and NSAIDs commonly used by migraineurs. The rare occurrence of surgical shock presents another potential dilemma that has already been discussed above; you may want to ask your doctor to start with small doses should sympathomimetic drugs become necessary in such a situation.

Dental Anesthetics*

Most of us are probably more familiar with dental anesthetics than we would like to be. Of course, we're grateful to be spared the pain that would otherwise accompany various dental procedures, but few exactly look forward to the injection itself or to the lingering numbness afterward. For us

*Labeled as risky for migraineurs on theoretical grounds, not yet supported by research or general concensus.

migraineurs there is a more serious concern, however. Many of us will develop attacks when the anesthetic wears off. Because this reaction may be delayed for up to 24 hours, we may not even connect it with the injection. And if symptoms occur sooner, we may blame the stress associated with the dental visit.

Once you understand the source of your symptoms, you can avoid, or at least greatly minimize, migraine reactions without sacrificing the pain relief that the anesthetic provides. In most cases the reaction stems not so much from the anesthetic itself as from a vasoconstrictor added to decrease the blood supply in the treated area. The purpose of this constrictor is two-fold: first to reduce bleeding during surgery, and secondly to keep the area numb longer. For nonsurgical work, such as filling cavities, neither action is necessary, but most dentists routinely include the ingredient anyway.

If you develop migraine symptoms after receiving dental anesthetics, your dentist probably will be willing to change his procedure once you explain your problem. I worked this out with mine so that I can enjoy needed pain relief for fillings without later symptoms by using the weakest solution (3%) of mepivacaine (usually sold as Carbocaine) and one without the customary vasoconstrictor, epinephrine. This formulation is shorter acting than the constrictor-containing solution, but I find that it lasts much longer than the predicted twenty to thirty minutes.

In the case of lengthier or bloodier work, a vasoconstrictor might be needed. In that case, I would take preventive medication, probably antihistamine, because some other good antimigraine drugs, such as aspirin and ibuprofen, tend to cause excessive bleeding during or after surgery. In any case it would be essential to get the dentist's approval before taking any medication. A primary concern would be avoiding any blood-thinning drugs until all danger of bleeding had passed.

Other Local Anesthetics*

Like dental anesthetics, other local anesthetics often contain vasoconstrictors and can therefore spell trouble for migraineurs. These chemicals are injected at the site prior to minor surgical procedures, and in cases involving the nose, throat, and larynx, vasoconstrictors are especially likely to be included. Once again, talk to your doctor in advance about whether there is actually any concern about bleeding during surgery or whether the use of a vasoconstrictor is simply routine and possibly unnecessary. Then the two of you can decide jointly how to proceed. Options include omitting the vasoconstrictor, lowering the dose, and/or taking migraine medication to forestall a possible reaction.

*Labeled as risky for migraineurs on theoretical grounds, not yet supported by research or general concensus.

Contrast Dyes

The dye Metrizamide (the medical term is "contrast medium") is injected into the spinal cord before brain X-rays (cerebral angiography), usually when physicians want a better view of suspicious areas that have shown up on scans. It is a well known medical fact that this chemical may cause migraine or at least severe migraine-like headache. Inform or remind the supervising physician of your migraine susceptibility if you must have this injection, and don't attempt to cut short the prescribed period of bedrest afterward. Lying still will help to avoid or minimize headache. (A different chemical is used for the contrast medium in MRIs—one that is generally free of side effects.)

Ulcer Medications

The widely used stomach-histamine blockers, cimetidine and ranitidine (usually sold as Tagamet and Zantac), both have been implicated as causes of headache in susceptible individuals. Of the two, Zantac reportedly causes less difficulty.

These popular drugs are also known to affect blood levels of other medications. Therefore it is particularly important to keep your doctor(s) informed about everything else you are taking as well as about any changes noticed in symptoms while using these acid-blocking agents.

Nonsteroidal Anti-Inflammatory Drugs (NSAIDs)

Many members of this drug family have proven effective in both preventing and interrupting migraine, but ironically at least one of them is known sometimes to cause or worsen headache. That drug is indomethacin, usually sold as Indocin. Most commonly used as an arthritis drug, Indocin may help cluster headache and several migraine variants (namely, ice-pick headache and headache associated with strenuous exercise or orgasm), but in at least some trials it has been shown to worsen other varieties of migraine. One source suggests that this NSAID sometimes is troublesome to migraineurs because it passes through the blood–brain barrier more readily than other drugs in this family.

Caffeine

This common vasoconstrictor appears in many over-the-counter and prescription pain and cold relief preparations, as well as in popular anti-drowsiness products. Anacin and Excedrin are just two of many such caffeine-containing medications. Some formulations of menstrual medications contain this stimulant as well. A regular-strength Anacin tablet contains 32 milligrams, and an Excedrin tablet has about twice that amount, as does Midol Extra Strength Menstrual Formula.

Caffeine can be helpful for halting a migraine attack, but its regular use should be avoided or restricted because headache may occur in susceptible people when the chemical's constricting effect wears off. Most migraine diets recommend no more than two daily 5-oz. servings of coffee or tea. (*See* Chapter 6 for more details about dietary caffeine.) Some sensitive migraineurs experience worsening of symptoms after taking in far less than that amount, however.

Thyroid Medication*

Use of supplementary thyroid hormones (Synthroid is a popular synthetic product) can initiate or aggravate symptoms if blood levels of the hormone become too high. This hormone has been shown to increase dietary amine sensitivity, already a frequent problem in migraine. Levels should be checked at least yearly, or sooner if migraine status worsens, by means of a blood test called a "complete thyroid profile."

Parkinson's Medications

Levodopa or carpidopa (usually sold as Sinemet and Dopar), used to treat Parkinson's disease, are known to worsen migraine. These drugs act to increase levels of the neurotransmitter dopamine in the brain and may cause an imbalance among brain chemicals.

Antidepressants

Two relatively new antidepressants, fluoxetine (Prozac) and trazodone (Deseryl), both of which also are used as migraine preventives, rather ironically are recognized as causing frequent though milder headaches in some patients. My personal experience suggests that too much Prozac (and presumably too high a resulting serotonin level) causes the headaches related to that particular medication. If you take Prozac, or one of its close cousins, Paxil (paroxetine) or Zoloft (sertraline), look for a level that controls migraine and/or depressive symptoms without provoking milder daily headaches. (It's possible that the trazodone-initiated headaches may be dose related as well.)

Sulfa and Codeine

These two very different medications—the first an antibiotic frequently used to treat urinary tract and some other infections, the second a narcotic used as a pain reliever and cough suppressant—are both extremely common

---

*Labeled as risky for migraineurs on theoretical grounds, not yet supported by research or general concensus.

allergens that can act as indirect migraine triggers. (In some states, over-the-counter cough syrups may contain codeine, making it possible for cold sufferers who are not careful label readers to be taking it without their knowledge.) Headache, nausea, and vomiting are frequent side effects of codeine; lightheadedness and dizziness also can occur. For sulfa, possible side effects are not only headache but also nausea, vomiting, dizziness, and ringing in the ears. These potential side effects are identical to the migraine symptoms of many sufferers. If you notice migraine symptoms worsening while taking either of these drugs, ask your doctor for an alternative.

Specifically known to worsen migraine symptoms is a synthetic sulfa-like antibacterial medication commonly used in treating urinary tract and ear infections, as well as travelers' diarrhea. This drug, trimethoprim-sulfamethoxazole, is available both as a generic and sold under various brand names, including Bactrim. When my doctor used to prescribe this artificial sulfa preparation to treat my urinary tract infections, I invariably wound up with a migraine within a day or two. At first I didn't realize what was happening and simply blamed my rotten feelings on the ailment itself. The trouble ceased after I finally caught on and asked to switch to a penicillin-like drug to treat the infections.

Disulfiram

Usually sold as Antabuse, this medication often is used as part of an alcohol treatment program. Taken once or twice a day, it reacts with any alcohol consumed to cause highly unpleasant and sometimes dangerous symptoms. Thus it provides extra motivation to avoid drinking. Regrettably this drug is known to initiate or increase migraine symptoms. Some evidence suggests that following a strict migraine diet may minimize this effect greatly.

Cocaine

This illegal narcotic is a vasoconstrictor that is known to cause or worsen migraine.

Sulfites

Used as preservatives in some over-the-counter and prescription medications, especially intravenous and spray preparations, this chemical family sometimes causes or worsens headache symptoms. Ironically (as previously mentioned), this additive commonly occurs in nebulized bronchodilator solutions for treating asthmatics, the very group that is most likely to suffer a serious reaction from it. However, metered-dose bronchodilator inhalers for asthma generally do *not* contain this troublesome chemical. Advise both your doctor and pharmacist if you are sensitive to this ingredient.

For information on the possible sulfite content of a particular medication, consult your pharmacist, the package insert that comes with the drug, or the PDR. Over-the-counter drug labels are not required to indicate the presence of inactive ingredients, but most manufacturers voluntarily list the entire product contents.

Do you notice a migraine reaction within 36 hours after eating large amounts of dried fruit preserved with sulfur dioxide? If so, you definitely should be cautious about sulfites in drugs. Reactions are often dose related, however. I am sensitive to sulfites in foods, but experience no reaction from my annual influenza inoculation, even though the serum label lists a tiny amount of the chemical as a preservative.

Cyclosporin

This immune system suppressant, sold as Sandimmune, is used to prevent rejection after organ transplant. Headache is but one of many unpleasant side effects associated with its use. Obviously in a life or death situation, such a price may well be worthwhile.

Lithium

Sold as Lithobid or Eskalith or under other brand names, this psychiatric drug is used to treat manic depression and some other illnesses, including even certain forms of cancer. It has been shown to help cluster headache, but in most trials it appears to worsen migraine (with the exception of one rare form of the disorder, i.e., cyclical migraine). Again, a hard choice may be involved for certain individuals who need this drug for psychiatric symptoms, but find that it worsens their headaches.

Antifungal Agents

Griseofulvin, a special antibiotic used for treating various fungal infections—such as ringworm, athlete's foot, and fungal conditions of the finger or toenail—is known to cause or worsen migraine in predisposed individuals. This drug is sold under several brand names, including Fulvicin and Grisactin.

Fertility Drugs

Clomiphene (Clomid/Serophene), given to women to stimulate ovulation and ultimately pregnancy, is known to cause headache as well. But rather ironically, in at least one man, this same drug given to increase a low sperm count resulted in near elimination of previously severe migraine headaches.

Vitamin A and Its Derivatives

Large amounts of this vitamin, taken as a food supplement, and its close cousin isotretinoin (Accutane), a popular treatment for severe cystic acne, are known to initiate or worsen headache symptoms. About 5% of Accutane patients complain of headache as a side effect.

Beta-carotene, the raw material for Vitamin A, is considered a safer supplement for people who are unable or unwilling to get sufficient Vitamin A from food sources, because the former does not build up in the system the way the pure form of the vitamin does. In the case of acne, Accutane probably should be reserved for very stubborn cases of the severe cystic form of the condition not responding to more conventional remedies such as antibiotics. If migraine symptoms begin or worsen while on this medication, of course you would want to discuss the situation with your physician. Some people may have to choose between the optimum treatment for their acne versus a more favorable headache scenario.

The Big Picture: *Nonheadache Medications*

In summary, migraine symptoms can be improved or worsened by medication taken as treatment for other disorders.

Migraineurs should approach the following drugs with caution:

- Vasodilators and vasoconstrictors
- Amphetamines and closely related medications given for weight control, narcolepsy, and hyperactivity
- Adrenaline-producing or releasing drugs, such as decongestants, given for colds and sinus problems, as well as medications commonly given or asthma and for allergic, surgical, or other forms of shock
- Anesthetics (general, dental, and local)
- The hormones estrogen and thyroid
- Drugs that lower blood sugar
- Drugs that deplete brain serotonin or increase other neurotransmitters

Other conditions usually can be treated successfully without adversely affecting migraine by choosing alternative drugs and/or by reducing the dosage of needed medications.

If you are uncertain about whether a medication you are taking belongs to one of these potentially troublesome classes, talk to your doctor or pharmacist and check the PDR in your public library. If you suffer from severe migraines and are concerned about minimizing or avoiding risky drugs in emergency situations, you may want to consider enrolling in Med-

Alert or a similar program and wearing a bracelet or necklace to provide medical warnings.

Balance to Be Achieved

To obtain effective relief from other medical conditions without aggravating migraine symptoms.

Chapter 10

Getting Effective Treatment

Benefit Versus Risk

The Magic Cure

It's probably safe to say there's not a migraineur alive who hasn't at least wished for a magic pill to cure the disorder. Most of us have actively sought such a remedy—some more frantically than others. Usually we have been at least somewhat disappointed in our search. For some sufferers, pursuing the magic cure will become a life-long preoccupation. For many others this quest will dramatically color, or perhaps even dominate, one or more decades of their lives. There's not much that a severe sufferer would not try in order to avoid or interrupt an attack: An acquaintance recently told me she had tried everything but witch doctors. In past years when narcotics were often prescribed for severe pain, addiction was not an uncommon occurrence among migraineurs seeking relief from their misery. Even today certain migraine-relieving drugs can lead either to dependence or to rebound headache, and indeed—at least in the long run—may create more problems than they solve.

"Any time you hear about many different drugs being touted for treating one particular illness, then you can assume that none of them is very effective," a Norfolk, Virginia, neurologist told me just a few years ago in reference to migraine medications. I wasn't sure I agreed with his logic at the time, but my subsequent experience has shown him to be at least partly right. Of course the same statement could be made concerning many other chronic illnesses, but it does illustrate the point that migraine is a very complex condition not yielding to any single, easy solution.

Like other drugs, every migraine medication does have its limits: None banishes all headaches; none works for every sufferer; and none is totally lacking in unpleasant side affects. As with any chronic illness, the trick in migraine treatment is to maximize benefits while minimizing both immediate and long-term discomfort and risk. That's the balance to be achieved in this particular quest: the best possible benefit-versus-risk profile. One reason I call achieving such a positive profile a "trick" is that finding the drug of choice is a highly individualized matter. To paraphrase Dr. Blau, Ms. Smith's headache is not Ms. Jones' headache—a truly profound bit of wisdom too often forgotten in the harried, everyday practice of medicine.

Medications are used to control migraines in two different, but often complimentary, ways—either as prophylactics to prevent an attack or as abortive agents to stop an attack in its initial stages. Each approach has its advantages and disadvantages. Most authorities advise reliance on abortive medication as long as attacks are contained episodes occurring no more than two or three times a month. If episodes are disabling or simply more frequent, however, and fail to respond to abortive medications, many recommend the use of a preventive drug—usually a beta-blocker, calcium channel blocker, or antidepressant. Additionally, other medications are frequently given to minimize pain and nausea and/or to sedate the miserable patient. Combination products are popular.

Guidelines for Choosing a Specific Medication

As medical consumers we can take specific steps to assure the most favorable benefit/risk ratio when choosing a new medication. Through careful research and thoughtful consideration of our individual situations, we can stack the odds in our favor. The following actions are appropriate in this regard:

1. Tell your prescribing physician every medication you already take, or are likely to take in the near future, including not only prescription drugs, but also over-the-counter preparations and even vitamins. (Some doctors wisely ask patients to bring in all medications for joint inspection and discussion. Surely, the physician who does not investigate current medications before suggesting new ones calls his competence into question.)
2. Advise your prescribing physician about all other diagnosed or suspected medical conditions, even if he doesn't ask. Tell him about significant family medical trends as well.
3. Read up on any suggested medication before you actually begin taking it. Doctors are busy people, and since they are only human, even they overlook pertinent factors on occasion. You may choose to conduct this independent research either before or after you discuss a particular treatment with your physician. You can find pertinent information in the *Physicians' Desk Reference* (hereafter abbreviated as PDR) available in

library reference sections, as well as in the package insert from the drug company. Most pharmacies will give you a free copy of such inserts if you simply tell them you are thinking about using the medication, and some offer their own patient advisory leaflets in addition. Just to be on the safe side, you may want to consult an independent third source, such as the *AARP Pharmacy Services Drug Handbook* or Joe Graedon's *People's Pharmacy* series, both of which are also in most public libraries. By then you should have a very good idea about whether or not the medication in question is appropriate for you.

4. If you do your research after receiving your prescription, don't hesitate to contact your doctor about any questions or concerns that may arise.

Migraine Drugs at a Glance

Appendix H gives you an overview of the most popular medications. If you are looking for concise information, you may decide to turn to it now. On the other hand, if you are interested in a more in-depth discussion about migraine drugs, then continue to read the body of this chapter. If you are unsure as to which course would be more helpful, then you might skim the following sections. (Of course, if you decide to skip or skim these detailed sections, you can always come back to them later, after reading the appendix.)

Migraine Abortive Agents: *A Stitch in Time...*
May Lead to More Serious Problems Down the Road

The most popular abortive agents are probably aspirin, butalbital combinations, ergot preparations, and Midrin, all of which are discussed below. In fairly recent controlled trials, another category of medications—the nonsteroidal anti-inflammatory drugs (NSAIDs)—has shown an impressive ability to interrupt attacks, but so far it doesn't seem to have caught on among practitioners involved in everyday migraine treatment.

The key to success in using all of the abortive agents mentioned so far, as any experienced migraineur probably already knows, is to take them early in an attack—well before any actual head pain begins. Those who are forewarned by specific sensory disturbances, such as the familiar visual aura, have little difficulty in using abortive medications successfully, at least initially. For that 85% of us who lack clearly defined signals of an impending attack, however, this early intervention presents a much greater challenge.

In additon, the risk from overusing abortive medication, especially ergot derivatives and barbiturates, but even ordinary analgesics such as aspirin and acetaminophen (Tylenol), is now widely recognized and cannot be overemphasized. All of these drugs, when used too frequently, often make symtoms worse instead of better. Those who have both full-fledged attacks and milder, more frequent headaches are at the greatest risk of developing chronic daily headache from the overuse of medication. (*See* the sections on "The Frustrating Quandary" on page 160 and "Reading Your Body's Signals" on page 161 for specific help with this problem.)

Later we will see how some of these problems can be minimized if the new migraine interrupter Imitrex fulfills its claim to stop an attack safely at any stage. First let's look at some of the advantages and disadvantages of the more traditional abortives.

Aspirin

Experience in British migraine clinics suggests that good old aspirin is a pretty effective way to stop many attacks. High initial doses are used, from 600–900 mg, to be repeated in 4–6 hours if needed; these doses must be taken early in the attack in order to be effective. For migraineurs with a sensitive stomach, or any type of gastrointestinal problem, such large doses of this gastric irritant would be unwise. Some sufferers can interrupt attacks with much smaller amounts, especially if caffeine is taken simultaneously, as in Excedrin. This, like many other dose requirements, seems to be an individual matter but, in general, larger doses are needed for interrupting a migraine attack than for ordinary pain control.

Nonsteroidal Anti-Inflammatories (NSAIDs)

These medications, some prescription and others available over-the-counter, are widely used in various pain syndromes—most notably arthritis. Like aspirin, they are anti-inflammatory agents as well as pain relievers. Both aspirin, the old standby migraine abortive, and the NSAIDs may owe their effectiveness to their ability to inhibit the production of prostaglandins, inflammatory chemicals that are present in many different organs and are implicated in migraine pain. Many migraineurs may be unaware that, as a class, NSAIDs are easier on the stomach than aspirin and probably can be used occasionally by most people without unpleasant or dangerous side effects. Additionally, some authorities believe that these newer medications interfere less with the body's natural pain-fighting mechanism than does their aspirin cousin, resulting in a more favorable long-term use profile.

NSAIDs are slowly but surely gaining in popularity as effective abortive medications. Some studies show that when used properly—early in the attack and in relatively large amounts—these medications can interrupt a migraine attack as effectively as ergot, but without the risk of nausea, rebound headache, and habituation associated with the older drug. One of the specific NSAIDs for which this claim is made is naproxen sodium (usually sold as Anaprox, but also available generically), which in one impressive study was given in an initial dose of 825 mg, an amount that effectively halted attacks in most sufferers tested. This drug, formerly available only by prescription, was released for over-the-counter sale (under the name Aleve) in early 1994. A more recent study shows the effectiveness of a similar drug, ibuprofen, available over-the-counter as Advil, Medipren, and Motrin, or as a less expensive store brand or generic version. In this trial comparing ibuprofen to a placebo (an inactive look-alike drug), subjects were given an initial oral dose of 800 mg and an additional 400 mg, if and when needed. The patients taking ibuprofen reported that their attacks were shorter and that they needed less supplementary pain medication than the ones getting just the placebo. No serious side effects were experienced.

One of the most recent studies using an NSAID concluded that injections of diclofenac sodium (usually sold as Voltaren) were exceptionally safe and effective in interrupting severe attacks. Eighty-eight percent of subjects given this treatment within 2–4 hours after the onset of their attacks obtained complete relief within 45 minutes; a few patients needed a second injection to completely halt symptoms during the 2–4 hour followup period. Side effects were mild and infrequent, according to the supervising physicians. Using the injectable form of an NSAID, as was done in this trial, reduces the risk of gastrointestinal irritation present with oral dosage and obviously offers more rapid absorption—two definite advantages.

For a time it appeared that the NSAID of choice in abortive treatment might well be a relatively new prescription medication called ketorolac (sold as Toradol). This drug, which has proven its effectiveness in controlled trials, is available in both oral and injectable forms. It often can stop a severe attack, once underway. And for convenient, fast relief, patients may learn to self-inject it at home for this purpose. Unfortunately the use of Toradol in Germany has recently been associated with a large number of cases of serious gastrointestinal bleeding and allergic reactions, causing the German Government to suspend its use, and leading some US physicians to reevaluate the drug. Ralph Nader's Public Citizen's Health Research Group now labels Toradol "DO NOT USE."

Regrettably, the only NSAID available in suppository form in this country is indomethacin (Indocin), the very one that is sometimes unsatisfactory in migraine control. That leaves the more cautious sufferer, who may need to avoid the new Imitrex as well as the controversial Toradol, with only the injectable Voltaren for fast migraine abortive use. Many of us may feel uncomfortable about giving our own injections, but like diabetics who have learned to inject their own insulin, we may find acquiring this skill to be in our long-term best interest.

Check with your doctor before trying any of these NSAIDs and read the package insert to be alerted for possible side effects ahead of time. The PDR lists several important contraindications (reasons for avoiding) for this class of drugs—most notably kidney or liver disease, aspirin allergy, and certain gastrointestinal disorders, as well as pregnancy. Ibuprofen may not be compatible with Inderal and certain other blood pressure medications. That and other NSAIDs may aggravate untreated or borderline high blood pressure. In order to protect the stomach, these medications should always be taken with food or milk, even though they are considerably less irritating than aspirin.

A personal note. As I mentioned earlier, I believe that NSAIDs are seriously underused by most doctors. I first learned about the drugs' use in migraine treatment from a sister migraineur who happened to be a medical insurance clerk; she was told about them by a drug salesman visiting the office where she worked. Of course, since she was unaware of the proper way to take the drugs, I did not learn that important information from her; neither, unfortunately, did I learn it from my doctor. Although my family practitioner was very cooperative about prescribing an NSAID for me when I requested it, he failed to tell me the importance of taking it very early and in a larger than normal dose. Perhaps that is the reason the drug failed to provide the hoped-for relief and I quickly abandoned it. Now that I am taking a preventive medication, the nonprescription ibuprofen works very nicely in interrupting my mild symptoms. I will probably never know whether or not the proper dosage of the nonprescription anti-inflammatory would have stopped my formerly severe attacks. But I do know that a number of other migraineurs with whom I have shared the good news about ibuprofen are reporting success in halting attacks with its use.

Butalbital Products

BAC

Usually sold as Fiorinal, this product combines butalbital, a potentially addictive barbiturate, with aspirin and caffeine. (Other brand names are Fiorgen, Isollyl, Lanorinal, and Marnal.) In addition to heavily sedating many users, this drug, by its very nature, tends to require greater and greater amounts to produce the same effect and therefore can easily lead to physical dependence and eventual addiction. Users also risk the potential drawbacks of codeine mentioned previously. Indeed, practitioners report a significant occurrence of addiction with this medication, sometimes even requiring medically supervised withdrawal. And for women who use birth control pills, another consideration is that butalbital has been implicated in reducing the contraceptive effectiveness of those drugs.

Butalbital with Acetaminophen and Caffeine

A close cousin of Fiorinal, this product, often sold as Fioricet, simply substitutes acetaminophen for aspirin; it is often recommended for aspirin-sensitive individuals. (Equivalents are Esgic and Repan.) This combination poses the risks associated with Fiorinal, as outlined above—simply minus the aspirin. Furthermore, heavy use of acetaminophen risks kidney damage while offering virtually nothing toward migraine relief. Fioricet is also available with codeine. The addition of codeine increases the risk of abuse from these combination products.

The use of the barbiturate butalbital in any form carries some risk of addiction, destruction of natural pain fighters, and rebound headache. Well-informed doctors are quite aware of these risks; some continue to prescribe these drugs anyway, while carefully limiting frequency of use and warning patients of the dangers. Unfortunately physicians who are not quite up-to-date on the migraine scene continue to use them rather casually and without the appropriate precautions. A friend of mine was given a prescription for unlimited refills with the very dangerous instruction to take "one tablet every 4 hours as needed for headaches."

Midrin

This combination product is frequently prescribed for interrupting mild to moderate attacks. It contains three ingredients: a vasoconstrictor, a mild pain reliever, and a mild antihistamine-like sedative. The pain reliever is acetaminophen (Tylenol), a drug that is relatively ineffective against migraine.

Midrin is usually well tolerated, but it can cause or worsen dizziness. The medical literature does not reflect a specific rebound problem with this drug, but such an occurrence would not be surprising because of the product's vasoconstrictive action. Sufferers are warned to avoid the drug when they are running a fever. I never used Midrin, probably because by the time I was properly diagnosed my symptoms were already too severe.

Dr. Sheftell and I have a difference of opinion about this drug. He finds it effective and well tolerated in many patients and believes that it generally is underprescribed in migraine treatment. I, on the other hand, am against the drug on theoretical grounds, mainly because it is a fixed combination of ingredients, not allowing for individual dosage variations and exposing the patient to some drugs that may not be needed at all. I regret that the vasoconstrictive chemical in Midrin is not available as a single agent in this country.

Ergot

For several decades the treatment of choice for stopping severe attacks has been ergot or various ergot derivatives and combinations. The substance seems to effect serotonin activity and it obviously constricts blood vessels. The important thing is that, if taken early enough, ergot preparations will interrupt the headache process in many migraineurs. Experience has shown that this relief does not come without a price, however—sometimes a very high one.

Ergot is available in the following forms: a traditional oral preparation, a sublingual tablet (to dissolve under the tongue), and a suppository. Combining it with caffeine (as in Wigraine or Cafergot) benefits many. Dr. Sheftell points out that the lesser known Wigraine tablet contains the same combination of ingredients as Cafergot, but is absorbed 15 times faster, a definite benefit in migraine treatment. He goes on to advise that people who feel overstimulated by the amount of caffeine in these tablets may be better served by using just part of a Cafergot suppository; he notices with his patients that often one-fourth to one-half of a suppository will do the trick and contribute much less of the stimulating caffeine. This can be a definite plus in migraine treatment because many sufferers resolve attacks by sleeping once the worst pain subsides.

Nausea is an extremely common side effect of ergot. For years in British migraine clinics, antinauseants have been given a few minutes before ergot and/or aspirin. This combination seems much less common in this country, but perhaps it should be used more frequently. Antinauseants are helpful not only in the obvious sense, that is, in preventing or stopping nausea, but also are important for another reason: It is widely recognized that intestinal absorption is decreased during an attack, thus rendering abortive and pain-relieving medications less effective. Antinauseants help to increase that intestinal absorption and thus aid the effectiveness of other medications.

Ergot is most effective when it is taken very early in an attack. I was told to take it at the very first sign of a impending headache. This requirement for early administration puts the sufferer in somewhat of a bind, however. The migraineur is advised to take ergot promptly—indeed before the possible severity of the attack can be judged—and yet usually is cautioned to take it no more than once or twice a week because of its potential for causing rebound headache and eventually setting up a cycle of daily pain. (There is one exception to this strict dosage limitation: the use of ergot derivatives for 3–5 days during the most vulnerable phase of the menstrual cycle is usually considered quite safe and effective.)

Most authorities warn patients to avoid taking ergot when they have a fever unless they first clear it with their physician. In addition to these usual cautions, Dr. Seymour Diamond, a leading US authority on headache, advises that ergot use is apt to be unsatisfactory for attacks lasting more than two hours. My experience confirms this warning; I only wish I had been aware of it years ago rather than learning about the drug's limitations the hard way.

I first used the sublingual ergot tablets. (These are not to be chewed or even sucked, but must simply be allowed to dissolve under the tongue.) I was told to lie down in a dark room for about an hour after using this medication, not very practical advice since I invariably threw up about a half hour later—just a minor inconvenience compared to the horrendous rebound headache I would then experience about 24 hours later. The actual head pain during those rebound episodes was worse than any I'd ever suffered, and totally unresponsive to any pain reliever. Not as bad as a full-fledged migraine attack—for these ergot-induced headaches lasted only a few miserable hours and were not accompanied by further nausea or other disabling symptoms—but still far short of the cure I was seeking. I have learned that my reaction to ergot was unusual; most people do not develop rebound headache from this drug unless they use it more than once or twice a week.

I had a slightly less painful, but still unsatisfactory, experience with Cafergot tablets. Although they did not bring nausea or rebound headaches, neither were they totally successful in shutting down my attacks. After taking the compound, I found that at least my symptoms decreased enough to allow continued functioning—a definite improvement over my untreated state. Reliance on this combination product periodically over the course of about 6 months, however, gradually resulted in diminished effectiveness so that eventually my attacks were merely postponed for about 24 hours. Sometimes even such a postponement proved to be a convenience and comfort of sort—at least I had some choice about when I would suffer, thus retaining some measure of control.

Finally the time came when my endurance wore thin, and I was no longer willing to settle for mere postponement. My attacks had become more severe, and I was ready to override my fear of regular daily medication and to begin a serious evaluation of preventive drugs. (More on that process later in this chapter. Meanwhile, let's continue our consideration of abortive agents.)

Because all ergot preparations, especially when misused, have the potential of creating as many problems as they solve, there is reason for concern, particularly if you are using ergot more than two days a week. If your headaches seem to be getting more frequent, you definitely should touch base with your doctor. Please don't ever try to stop the habitual use of ergot on your own. Such a withdrawal requires medical supervision. Sometimes a preventive medication is required to take the place of ergot—or in really extreme cases, the habituated patient must be hospitalized and given a weaning medication on a temporary basis. In-patient headache clinics claim expertise in this ergot-withdrawal process.

Sumatriptan: Wonder Drug or Just Another Tool?

Both migraineurs and the medical community have eagerly welcomed the promising new drug sumatriptan (sold as Imitrex), approved by the FDA for use in this country in March, 1993. An impressively large study that included 1104 patients at 61 US medical sites shows treatment of acute migraine with injected sumatriptan to be highly effective and without serious side effects in relieving symptoms of the severe attack. In this hopeful study 70% of the subjects obtained total relief while experiencing only minor side effects from the drug—symptoms including tingling, dizziness, hot flashes, and injection-site reactions.

Sumatriptan may be more selective than ergot in constricting blood vessels outside the head, where such vasoconstriction is undesirable—particularly in the heart and the gastrointestinal tract. Both ergot and sumatriptan mimic brain serotonin activity—lending further support to the theory of serotonin deficiency as the basic cause of migraine.

According to the manufacturer, Cerenex Pharmaceuticals (a division of Glaxo, Inc.), Imitrex offers the following benefits to the patient experiencing a severe migraine attack: It allows simple, convenient at-home dosing; is highly effective whether given early or late in an attack; works quickly (pain usually begins to subside within 10 minutes and most patients experience significant improvement within 45 minutes); is nonsedating and usually restores the patient's ability to work; relieves all symptoms of the attack, including nausea and light sensitivity, as well as head pain; is equally effective in interrupting migraine either with or without aura; and can be used safely with most other medications (except with ergot and DHE taken during the previous 24 hours). If relief is obtained after the first injection, but the headache recurs, patients may repeat the treatment in two hours. In one trial of 235 patients, 31% needed a second dose.

Cerenex provides an instructional video, available through doctors and pharmacies, that explains exactly how to load, use, and care for the auto-injector, which the patient can use to self-administer the drug. (The starter kit itself contains an instructional leaflet for patients who don't own a VCR or who simply prefer getting their directions the old fashioned way.) The auto-injector is a spring-loaded device similar to the ones now used by medical personnel to prick the finger when drawing a small blood sample. No special medical skills are needed to use this device. The patient simply loads it and then pushes a button to inject the Imitrex liquid into her upper arm or thigh. The actual entry of the needle is not seen. My local pharmacist quotes a price, as of this writing, of $67.09 for a starter kit containing the auto-injector device and two syringes; two syringes only (as a refill) retail here for $63.29. (Some people are complaining that this price seems excessive, but I would have paid it in a heartbeat to stop one of my previously severe attacks.) Currently available in this country only for injections, Imitrex is expected to be released in an oral form soon.

Canadian doctors and their patients report largely favorable results after several years of experience with sumatriptan, but some cautious specialists have continued to point out that relatively little is known about this medication's potential for long-term side effects. Some also voice a concern about the short life of the drug, possibly necessitating repeat doses for patients whose attacks last for more than a few hours and perhaps even leading to rebound headaches, similar to those seen with caffeine and ergot. Indeed in April, 1993, a Canadian physician reported on three patients who appeared to develop rebound headaches after appropriately using this drug to relieve classical migraine attacks. He calls for further evaluation to determine the extent to which sumatriptan may cause rebound pain and a reexamination of the dosing guidelines as well.

Research has not established the safety of Imitrex for use in pregnant or nursing women. It is already recognized, however, that the drug is not appropriate for certain heart and blood pressure patients and should be used only with caution in those with reduced kidney or liver function. In patients with certain risk factors, the first dose should be administered under supervision in the doctors' office. This precaution is in order for postmenopausal women, those with a family history of heart disease, and those who are overweight, have high cholesterol, smoke, or do not exercise regularly. Patients with any of these risk factors should receive both an electrocardiogram and a blood pressure check 15 minutes after the sumatriptan injection.

Dr. Sheftell notes that most of his patients who have tried this new drug are very enthusiastic about it. Many of them, who have used numerous other medications in attempts to interrupt their attacks, find Imitrex far superior to their previous treatments. Frequently they are able to return to work in a very short time after receiving the medication, showing dramatic improvement from very debilitating symptoms.

It may very well be that Imitrex proves to be a boon for sufferers of the occasional but severe attack, but we must wait to see whether the drug lives up to its promise of effective, and truly safe, relief.

Pain Relievers (Analgesics) and Sedatives: *Friends or Enemies?*

Migraine pain is recognized as being both severe and particularly stubborn. Once the headache phase of an attack begins, the pain generally is not responsive to standard analgesics. Like most sufferers, you have probably experienced firsthand exactly what that nonresponsiveness means—*Pain, Pain, and More Pain,* sometimes lasting for days. Many authorities believe that a faulty natural pain control system is at least partly responsible for the disorder we call migraine. Additionally, research has shown that changes occurring in the stomach early in an attack lead to decreased absorption of medications. Those two factors may explain our generally poor response to pain medications. Some British practitioners prefer using effervescent aspirin in migraine treatment, believing it is better absorbed than the regular tablets. In British migraine clinics, antinauseants are also routinely administered prior to the aspirin or other analgesic. Unfortunately, domperidome, the antinauseant used in many other countries, is not yet available in the United States, and those antinauseants available here seem either much less effective or potentially more dangerous. Reglan, the abortive agent discussed in the previous section, also acts as an effective antinauseant, but carries some potential for dangerous, or at least unpleasant, reactions. Dr. Sheftell advises that this risk is less with oral dosing, however, and points out as well that an over-the-counter drug called Emetrol is a fairly effective and extremely safe antinauseant.

Many experts believe that frequent use of analgesics may further weaken an already malfunctioning pain control system, leading to a vicious cycle of more attacks and more need for medication. Likewise, they hold that the regular use of pain relievers is counterproductive for those on preventive medications, because it actually interferes with the effectiveness of those drugs. For those who have become caught up in this vicious cycle of daily analgesic use, it is thought that a period of about 8–12 weeks without such medication is required to allow the natural pain control system to rejuvenate. In extreme cases, special medical treatment may be required during this analgesic withdrawal period. Seizures have been known to occur—particularly with butalbital, the commonly prescribed barbiturate. There seems to be a difference of opinion about whether or not NSAIDs, like many other analgesics, interfere with this natural pain control mechanism. Perhaps this controversy exists because they are a relatively new family of drugs, only recently used in headache treatment.

Over-the-Counter Remedies

If an attack is not halted before the headache phase, various drugs are frequently taken for pain relief and/or sedation. For example, migraineurs continue to use traditional analgesics, such as acetaminophen, plain aspirin, and now the newer NSAIDs in attempts to relieve their painful symptoms, but most admit that such use is much like putting a finger in the dike to hold back the flood. Indeed, the former is no match for migraine, and unless the latter agents are taken very early in the attack, and usually in larger-than-normal doses, even they seldom work. Physicians often fail to emphasize these conditions.

Prescription Remedies

Acetaminophen with Codeine (Tylenol 2, 3, and 4)

Although often recommended, this is probably not a good choice for migraine pain for two reasons. First, acetaminophen (the generic name for Tylenol) is not an anti-inflamatory, and therefore is relatively ineffective against headache pain. Second, codeine is a common allergen that provokes nausea and vomiting in many patients—not exactly welcome among migraineurs. Furthermore, codeine is both extremely constipating and potentially addictive.

Butorphanol Tartrate Nasal Spray (Stadol NS)

A new weapon in the migraine arsenal, this metered nasal spray begins working against pain in as little as 15 minutes and lasts between four and six hours, on average. As a member of the opiate family, the drug has some potential for abuse and addiction in long-term users (according to the PDR), although probably less so than some of the older narcotics. It often causes drowsiness and dizziness, as well as nausea and vomiting, and has a high potential for interacting with other drugs, including antihistamines and alcohol. Nevertheless Stadol may be helpful for sufferers of severe, but occasional, attacks (especially if head pain is the primary symptom) since it allows for convenient at-home administration without needles.

Tranquilizers

The lucky migraineur is able to sleep through attacks naturally, but those of us who are not so fortunate have endured many long nights of sleepless misery. Some authorities suggest giving a single dose of a short-acting tranquilizer, such as lorazepam (usually sold as Ativan), to promote sleep during a severe attack. Of course, these drugs are potentially addictive, but occasional use is probably safe for most people. Those who have trouble handling alcohol or have a family history of alcohol or drug abuse might be wise to avoid them, however.

The Frustrating Quandary: *Should I Reach for That Bottle?*

The notoriously poor response migraineurs get from pain relievers, once an attack is underway, underscores the desirability for early detection and treatment. If your early symptoms fail to signal the difference between severe attacks and milder headaches, you may find yourself in somewhat of a bind in this regard, however. One extreme is to become jumpy and overreactive, taking abortive medication at every twinge and thus risking habituation and rebound headache. Another, probably more common, response is ignoring or failing to tune into subtle clues provided by our bodies—perhaps even denying or attempting to wish away an impending attack. Migraineurs frequently make frustrating comments, such as, "How can I tell whether it's really going to be a migraine or just a regular headache?" (Or, perhaps better put, in light of recent research findings, "How can I tell whether it's going to be a really severe headache or just an average one?") With good reason, most of us are reluctant to take medications unnecessarily and therefore tend to postpone them until it's too late. Finding the prudent middle ground is a real challenge.

So that sufferers can medicate appropriately, Dr. Sheftell recommends that we learn to think of our headaches as occurring in stages. (This is particularly important for those of us who have mixed headache syndrome, for we are the most likely to overuse medication.) Here is the way he outlines his system: If symptoms are very mild—resulting in nothing more than foggy thinking—simply ignore them. If, however, they progress to the annoying stage and begin to interrupt normal activity, then consider an appropriate dose of an NSAID or Midrin (unless there are medical reasons to avoid these drugs). Only if the head actually begins to throb, or if other clear signs of migraine are present (nausea or light sensitivity, for example) should a stronger drug be considered. If the NSAID or Midrin fails to halt the attack, then ergot or sumatriptan may be appropriate.

At this point two Wigraine or Cafergot tablets can be taken. If symptoms continue, the Wigraine or Cafergot dose can be repeated in one hour. If nausea tends to be a problem or if ergot has failed to provide relief in the past, an oral antinauseant can be taken 15–30 minutes before the ergot combination; and if severe nausea prevents oral medication, then both an antinauseant and abortive can be taken in suppository form (one-fourth to one suppository to start). Again, if symptoms persist after an hour, this dose can be repeated.

Sumatriptan, rapidly becoming a popular alternative to ergot, does not require an antinauseant. In fact this new drug not only causes less nausea than ergot does, but it sometimes even decreases that disabling symptom while relieving head pain and other accompanying miseries. In contrast to ergot, however, a second dose of sumatriptan should be taken (after 2 hours) if and only if partial relief has already been experienced.

Such a cautious, systematic approach to migraine pain should bring appropriate relief for many, while minimizing the possibility of overdosing.

Reading Your Body's Signals: *Identifying Your Prodrome*

Researchers have discovered that in many migraineurs at least some attacks are preceded by significant changes in mood, sensory perception, energy level, or appetite. These bodily warning signs may occur all the way from 24 hours to just a half hour before the onset of the attack and may be either rather subtle or quite pronounced. According to British expert Dr. J. N. Blau, on average these symptoms appear about three hours before the headache.

The medical term for this constellation of symptoms and/or the time period during which it appears is "prodrome." Sometimes intimates will be aware of the changes even before the sufferer. The rather obvious advantage to tuning into these signals is that such an awareness gives the sufferer an opportunity to stop the expected attack. This is particularly valuable information for the person who has only full-fledged attacks and is thus in much less danger of overusing medication. Such a person may wish to put biofeedback or other relaxation skills to work at this stage, either instead of, or in addition to, more traditional remedies. An obvious plus for the latter choice is that overuse poses no physical dangers.

Examples of signs occurring during the prodrome might be dizziness, lightheadedness, numbness anywhere in the body—perhaps around the lips, for instance—sensitivity to light, odors, or sound, or a "closed head" syndrome—that is, a hearing distortion resulting in the perception that the person's own voice is coming from the bottom of a barrel. Mood and/or energy levels may be either unexplainably very high or very low, while appetite may either lessen or increase to an unusual degree. Specific food cravings may be involved. Other prodromal symptoms that have been reported are varied and include such things as excessive yawning, tearing, sneezing, and nausea. In short, prodromal experiences are strikingly like aura experiences, except they usually are more subtle and prolonged. Scientists interpret these prodromal signs as indications that a portion of the brain called the hypothalamus is involved in the origin of the migraine attack. The hypothalamus, located directly behind the eyes, acts as a kind of master switchboard for many different bodily functions, including appetite, mood, and blood vessel tone.

There seems to be some confusion about cause and effect in this situation—both among experts and sufferers themselves. For instance, is fatigue an actual trigger of an attack or is it merely a prodromal signal that an attack is on its way? Current knowledge does not yet allow us to answer that question. Furthermore, in female sufferers, hormone fluctuations may actually be responsible for some of these bodily changes, and those fluctuations in turn may trigger the attack. Whatever the exact scenario, the individual sufferer will benefit from learning to recognize her prodrome, if any, and to use appropriate remedies very early when they are apt to be the most effective.

Sufferers often dismiss these warning signs entirely or at least fail to connect them with a brewing attack. The headache diary provides an effective method for learning to recognize your own prodromal signs, and the 24-hour backtracking method of keeping such a diary is usually effective without being unduly burdensome. At the time of your next attack, as soon as the worst symptoms subside, record any unusual physical or emotional symptoms you experienced during the 24 hours prior to the actual headache. Get help from your family and/or close associates in identifying these signs. Continue to record this information for several months, reviewing and mulling over your entries from time to time. Soon you may be able to identify a pattern—one, or perhaps several, signs that occur before some or all of your attacks.

In my case, I usually notice unusually intense hunger coupled with unexplained fatigue about three hours before the onset of any actual headache symptoms. In my premedication days, the first sign was usually a headrush (a sudden feeling of blood rushing to the head), but I rarely experience that now.

Emergency Treatment: *Relief for the Debilitating Attack*

It's a relatively common occurrence for migraineurs to seek emergency treatment. When we fail to take our at-home medications in time, or for some reason they are not effective, we may be left with severe pain and nausea that completely prevent normal functioning. Such an experience is much more likely to occur in a migraineur who is neither taking a preventive medication nor following a precautionary lifestyle regimen.

In severe cases, disabling symptoms can persist for several days or even longer. The medical term for such a severe, prolonged attack is "status migraine." According to experts, most of these status attacks result from the abuse of ergot or narcotic medications. In these attacks, when nausea and vomiting often prevent intake and/or retention even of liquids, dehydration sometimes occurs. In such instances, intravenous fluids may be given, and if the attack is continuing when the migraineur seeks treatment, dihydroergotamine (DHE-45) often is given along with the fluids. It is considered the drug of choice for interrupting the severe attack once underway. Although DHE is related to ergot as its name suggests, this drug is chemically different from other ergot derivatives. Most significantly, DHE is less likely to cause rebound headache than are other ergot drugs.

Although DHE is considered a very safe drug, there is some controversy among different medical specialities about its effectiveness and the way the drug should be used—whether alone or in combination with an antinauseant. Generally, headache specialists view DHE very positively (and traditionally many routinely have given it along with an antinauseant medication), whereas some emergency-room physicians, often involved in treating headache patients, have a less favorable view. Two controlled studies published by emergency-room physicians in 1990 call DHEs effectiveness into question, specifically raising the issue of whether it actually is the agent responsible for interrupting the severe attack, as has long been held, or whether either Reglan or Compazine—the antinauseants frequently used *with* DHE—may in fact, be responsible for the improvement seen in treated patients. (At any rate, each of these latter drugs used alone appears to be much more effective than the narcotics popular in the past.)

One of my favorite doctors tells me that he considers these prescription antinauseants too dangerous for use in migraine treatment, but then he admittedly has never had a migraine, let alone a severe one. Troublesome side effects, such as muscle jerking and even seizures, although theoretically possible, are rarely experienced as a result of these drugs, when they are administered correctly. Indeed experience with Reglan in British migraine clinics testifies to its relative safety. Furthermore, the 1991 PDR claims that any unpleasant reactions can be halted with the injection of the common antihistamine, Benadryl. Dr. Sheftell advises that he and Dr. Rapoport frequently recommend Reglan to their patients. They use small doses (beginning with 5 mg) when the drug is given intravenously in status migraine, carefully monitoring patients for any signs of adverse reactions. And they go on to give DHE *only if* satisfactory relief is not obtained from the Reglan administration alone.

If you have received either DHE, Compazine, or Reglan, or are offered one of them in the future, surely you will want to discuss their risks and effectiveness with your doctor. You might well decide that the automatic joint use of an antinauseant with DHE is inappropriate since either drug is often quite effective alone. Such a combination, common though it is, may violate a basic rule of medical practice: Do not increase exposure and thus potential risk without a corresponding increase in benefits. We're right back to our benefit/risk equation again.

Interestingly, in a study published this year in which 38 headache specialists treated 311 migraine patients with DHE, the doctors concluded that the administration of an antinauseant was usually not necessary. DHE alone proved quite effective in interrupting the severe attack.

If Imitrex lives up to its promise for safe, effective at-home treatment during any phase of an attack, the need for these other emergency medications may be a thing of the past for most sufferers, and we will no longer need to concern ourselves with these very real issues of safety and efficacy involved with their use.

Better Safe Than Sorry: Precautions for Emergency Treatment

Because a few patients have tended to abuse some of the abortive and pain-relieving medications, doctors may be reluctant to provide emergency treatment unless they know the patient personally or the patient's physician has left a standing order. It may be wise to speak to your doctor about such a situation in advance, in case you ever find yourself needing this type of treatment when he is not available. Asking for a standing order for abortive drug care in a convenient hospital emergency room or walk-in clinic makes sense for someone who has had one or more severe attacks. Equally prudent would be a request for advance arrangements in case of out-of-town travel. When you leave town, at the very least carry with you the name, address, and telephone number of your primary-care physician—preferably in the form of a business card—so that unfamiliar doctors may contact him for information about your treatment.

Preventive Treatments: What Should We Do With the Corpse?

The way preventive medication is used in migraine treatment reminds me of the old joke in which the operation is judged to be a success even though the patient dies. Sometimes the drugs prescribed for us are quite effective in minimizing our primary symptoms, but the side effects they cause may be nearly as troublesome, or perhaps even more so, than our original complaints. Here's the bottom line: Unless overall well-being is enhanced by a particular medication, then treatment is a failure.

Another disturbing trend is that some physicians seem to rely more on the reports of drug performance in controlled research trials than on personal feedback from patients about a medication's effects. Research studies are extremely helpful, but they seldom tell the whole story—even when they are well designed and carried out—which is not always the case.

In order to keep our perspective about the necessity for lifestyle changes to complement any medication, it's important to remember that propranolol, the most effective migraine preventive in clinical trials, is at best no more than 50% effective in reducing the frequency and severity of attacks. And indeed, only about 70% of sufferers who take this medication experience any notable improvement.

If your attacks are significantly interfering with your life, it may be time to consider taking a preventive medication. (With the benefit of hindsight, I now regret having waited so long to take that step.) To gain a clearer perspective on this important decision, complete the personal work sheet in Appendix G. This work sheet reflects my basic philosophy about the role of medication in chronic illness: That is, that drug treatment should be kept as a last resort, to be used only if nondrug strategies fail to bring relief, and then only in conjunction with holistic lifestyle changes. Sharing the completed worksheet with your doctor would provide him with a comprehensive overview of your situation; and there's something almost magic about seeing the whole scenario spelled out in writing—both for you and for him.

Popular Preventives

As mentioned before, the most popular drug families used to prevent migraines are beta blockers, calcium channel blockers, and antidepressants. All three families have demonstrated some degree of effectiveness in controlled trials. A specific choice should be made chiefly on the basis of a thorough understanding of the individual patient's other medical conditions, with the goal of avoiding unpleasant or dangerous side effects and interactions with other medications.

Several drugs in each of these families have been shown in clinical trials to be effective in reducing both the frequency and severity of migraine symptoms. These drugs must be taken on a daily or more frequent basis. Of all the preventives in use, only three—the beta blockers propranolol (usually sold as Inderal) and timolol (sold as Blocadren) and the serotonin blocker methysergide (sold as Sansert) have received FDA approval for that specific purpose. The other individual drugs from these three families (as well as a few miscellaneous others that are being prescribed as migraine preventives) have proven safety records (at least to FDA satisfaction), but their effectiveness has been certified only for disorders *other than migraine*. Actually Sansert, the first drug to receive official FDA approval as a migraine preventive, is seldom used since other options have become available, because of its potential for serious side effects (most notably, rare but dangerous scar tissue formation in the chest or abdominal cavities).

The discussion of preventive drugs in the following section is not intended to be a comprehensive pharmaceutical review. Instead it is designed to point out some facts and opinions not usually presented in routine drug references and other headache books.

Beta Blockers

The discovery that this drug family, first developed for control of certain heart and blood pressure conditions, could be helpful in preventing migraine as well, was made entirely by accident. Now generally considered the first line of defense in migraine prevention, propranolol (Inderal) often is given in the form of Inderal LA (long acting)—a version of the drug that is especially convenient because it has to be taken only once a day.

Researchers tell us that about 70% of migraineurs who take Inderal obtain significant relief. Even today the exact mechanism by which Inderal and related drugs prevent headache is not well understood, but we do know that they prevent blood vessels from expanding and that this action can pose serious problems for certain individuals, including many migraineurs. The most compelling reason for avoiding these drugs is asthma. Less well known is that they often worsen any allergic symptoms or tendencies.

In addition, the beta blockers can cause especially troublesome side effects for individuals who suffer from poor circulation in the hands and feet. An acquaintance whose migraines were greatly helped by Inderal decided to discontinue the drug when she no longer was able to use her hands for simple daily tasks, like writing and chopping vegetables. There is, in fact, a higher than average rate of Raynaud's Syndrome among migraineurs. (Raynaud's is a blood vessel disorder that restricts circulation in the hands and feet.) Even if you have not received such a formal diagnosis, you may be risking trouble from restricted circulation by using a beta blocker. Of course this particular side effect is one that would be quite obvious and show up relatively quickly.

A similar, but more serious, concern about the action of beta blockers on blood vessels stems from the possible interference with the brain's blood supply. Some authorities feel this possibility poses an unacceptable danger for migraineurs, who, as a group, already have a significantly elevated risk of stroke—double that of the average person, according to data from the prestigious Physicians' Health study released in late 1991. All beta blockers interfere with cardiovascular fitness, and many users notice a decreased tolerance for exercise—an event that may not bode well for the stroke-prone patient.

Another drawback to long-term use is the fact that most, if not all, of the betas seem to cause an undesirable change in blood fats, including increased triglycerides and decreased levels of good cholesterol. As if this isn't enough to worry about, some authorities have expressed still another concern with long-term use of these medications, noting a need for gradually increased dosage to control migraine symptoms—and thus potential for an increased risk of undesirable reactions.

In addition, patients taking Inderal commonly complain of central nervous system symptoms like fatigue, sleep disturbances, and either the onset or worsening of depression. Because depressive tendencies are extraordinarily common among migraineurs, that particular side effect probably poses an especially serious threat to many of us.

To look at the other side of the coin, taking a beta blocker for migraine control might well be appropriate for a sufferer with high blood pressure that can't be controlled with lifestyle changes. In that case, there's a very good possibility that the same drug would control both conditions. Another plus for the beta blockers is that they frequently reduce symptoms of anxiety, especially nervousness in social situations. They also often are recommended as the treatment of choice for sufferers bothered with mitral valve prolapse, a condition seemingly quite prevalent among migraineurs.

Some of the side effects associated with Inderal can be minimized by using one of the newer beta blockers. To lessen symptoms of circulatory or respiratory constriction, you might consider metoprolol (Lopressor) or atenolol (Tenormin), both of which are also effective migraine preventives, although perhaps slightly less so than the more troublesome propranolol (Inderal). These newer drugs, at least when used in moderate doses—no more than 200 mg a day—are somewhat less troublesome for asthmatics, for example, and probably for those with poor circulation in the hands and feet as well. To minimize drowsiness and depression along with other central nervous system side effects associated with Inderal—namely sleep disturbances, sexual problems, confusion, and memory loss—one would want to select a drug that does not cross the blood–brain barrier as easily as Inderal. Atenolol (Tenormin) and nadolol (Corgard) fill the bill in that regard. Atenolol, then, is the only one of these medications that minimizes both circulatory and central nervous system side effects associated with this drug family.

In order further to minimize sleep disturbances, some practitioners advise taking beta blockers in the morning. You may have some leeway in dosage as well. Consider asking your doctor about supervising a dosage reduction in an effort to reduce any troublesome side effects.

Many drug manuals warn against sudden reduction or elimination of these medications. Dangerous heart rhythm disturbances can occur if dosage is changed abruptly.

Calcium Channel Blockers

Several different medications from this family have demonstrated some effectiveness as migraine preventives, and, until quite recently, seemed to be gaining in popularity. Verapamil (sold as Calan or Isoptin) is probably the most widely used in this country and seems to be well tolerated, with constipation the most commonly reported side effect. Like the betas, these drugs originally were developed as heart and blood pressure medications. Some of them, notably verapamil and diltiazem (sold as Cardizem), slow heart action and therefore should be avoided by people with congestive heart failure or advanced heart block. As is the case with their cousins the beta blockers, these drugs work in a rather mysterious way to control headaches. There is one basic and very significant difference between the two families, however. Instead of preventing blood vessel expansion as do the betas, these drugs actually prevent constriction, thus avoiding some of the dangerous or troublesome side effects caused by the former class of medications. Migraineurs with asthma or restricted circulation in the hands and feet, for example, are likely to tolerate these medications, whereas the betas would worsen those conditions. You can rest assured that these drugs do not interfere with calcium absorption and use in the teeth, bones, or other areas where the nutrient is essential, but only with the way calcium is used in muscle cells.

Recent results from the first large-scale controlled tests of two of these drugs, nifedipine (Procardia) and nimodipine (Nimotop), were quite disappointing. In fact, in some of the trials these medications appeared to be no more effective than placebos in preventing attacks. In spite of the fact that the effectiveness of these calcium blockers has not been well supported in controlled trials, individual sufferers continue to report obtaining good results with minimal side effects while taking some of these drugs.

The following points are worth keeping in mind if you decide to try a calcium blocker: Expect to wait up to two months before obtaining maximum benefits; minimize side effects by starting with small doses and gradually increasing them as necessary; and, if you experience irritating daily headache as a side effect, but are otherwise satisfied with your medication, you might want to consider asking your doctor either to reduce your dose, to switch to a different drug in the same family, or to prescribe a timed-release form of the drug. One interesting study shows that small doses of verapamil, 80 mg, twice a day, are nearly as effective as traditionally larger doses in preventing migraine. Nifedipine (Procardia), nicardipine (Cardene), and nimodipine (Nimotop) seem to be particularly likely to result in daily head-ache. And whereas verapamil has been more widely studied and used in this role, diltiazem has the lowest vasodilating action—a possible advantage for headache sufferers.

Some authorities are touting a new and radically different member of this drug family, flunarizine, which is already a popular migraine preventive in some countries and is currently under investigation by the FDA. Certain experts expect this drug to win quick approval for US use and to gain wide acceptance among migraineurs because of both its effectiveness and the convenience of its once-a-day administration. This drug does not lower blood pressure as do other calcium blockers—a plus for some patients, but an obvious drawback for others.

In one interesting trial of this new calcium blocker, 149 sufferers of common migraine were assigned to 16-week treatment with either flunarizine or the beta blocker metoprolol (Lopressor), a drug with proven effectiveness as a migraine preventive. In this Danish study these two drugs demonstrated equal effectiveness in minimizing headache frequency and severity, but a higher number of flunarizine-treated subjects discontinued treatment because of adverse side effects than did members of the metoprolol group. Depression and weight gain were cited by the majority of flunarizine subjects who dropped out. Metoprolol patients more often complained of gastro-intestinal symptoms, sleep disturbances, and muscle fatigue. The supervising neurologists judged depression to be the most serious side effect overall, with 8% of the flunarazine patients and 3% of the metoprolol patients developing that disorder for the first time. Daytime drowsiness was a frequent complaint initially, but that symptom subsided in both groups after the first few months of treatment.

An even more recent study has shown that adverse side effects from flunarazine can be greatly minimized (while still maintaining treatment effectiveness) by simply reducing the dose of the drug.

Antidepressants: Helpful Drugs

Antidepressants have proven themselves to be effective migraine preventives both in numerous controlled trials and in practical use. The tricyclic class of antidepressants—specifically amitriptyline (usually sold as Elavil or Endep), nortriptyline (usually sold as Pamelor), or doxepin (usually sold as Adapin or Sinequan)—has shown itself to be just slightly less effective than the beta blockers, but somewhat more effective than the calcium blockers in migraine treatment. But—and this is an important qualification—

because these antidepressants frequently are effective in very low doses, indeed significantly lower than those prescribed for depression, it is often possible to use them with minimal side effects. We migraineurs don't seem to be taking advantage of this opportunity for relatively untroubled relief, however. Perhaps doctors are reluctant to suggest antidepressants because of a lingering fear and misunderstanding among the general public concerning these drugs. Actually, knowledge seems to be somewhat scanty, both among doctors and patients, about the role these drugs play in relieving chronic pain syndromes, as well as about certain other qualities of the drugs.

Let me share with you some significant facts about this important class of migraine preventives: All antidepressants work on the brain's neurotransmitter system, designed to keep both serotonin and noradrenaline, or serotonin alone, available at the nerve terminals. These drugs are neither habit forming nor addictive; in fact they do not even change the mood of a "normal" person—someone not suffering from a mood disorder. In afflicted individuals, however, they do relieve mood disorders, such as depression and anxiety, as well as obsessive–compulsive tendencies. They are commonly prescribed for such diverse nonmood conditions as chronic pain occurring after shingles, and even for bed wetting. Some studies show that they relieve premenstrual symptoms as well.

The use of antidepressants in migraine treatment seems highly appropriate because their action is very straightforward. Scientists actually understand how and why they relieve headaches, unlike some other medications commonly used in migraine prevention. Research shows that the drugs' ability to relieve migraine is independent of their effect on mood. They also seem to be the migraine preventive most compatible with the use of biofeedback or other relaxation skills, presumably because they do not directly alter blood vessel tone, as do both categories of blockers.

In spite of the proven success and straightforward action of these drugs, however, migraineurs tend to approach them with great hesitancy and fear. Please remember these points: Antidepressants are effective migraine preventives, are nonaddictive, and do not alter mood in normal people. If your doctor suggests a trial of one of these drugs, there's definitely no implication that your headaches are psychological in origin.

Help for the Depressed

As Chapter 8 points out, there is a very strong link between depression and migraine, with some studies showing that as many as 40% of migraineurs suffer from the biologically determined, inherited form of the mood disorder (Chapter 11 further discusses this relationship.) Sometimes neither the migraineur nor the doctor is aware that the sufferer's low moods signify the presence of another illness, one that might have been suffered on and off through a lifetime and so might have come to be regarded as normal. If you suspect that you may be among the large number of migraineurs who are also depressed, it would probably be worth your while to have your symptoms evaluated by a psychiatrist, the specialist with the greatest expertise in diagnosing and treating this disorder. If you do decide to see such a specialist, be sure to report that you suffer from migraine. And, of course, if you do have tendencies toward depression or have a strong family history of the disorder, it makes even more sense to consider an antidepressant as your migraine preventive of choice. It's a sensible way to kill two birds with one stone.

Choice of a Particular Antidepressant

Although amitriptyline (Elavil) seems to be the member of this family with the best record in headache control—possibly because it is one of the oldest tricyclics and has simply been tested the most—it probably is responsible for the worst side effects as well, sometimes even at relatively low doses. (It has the greatest drying effects and potentially can cause the most troublesome heart rhythm disturbances.) In order to minimize side effects, many experts recommend starting with the lowest possible dose of a newer antidepressant with a more favorable treatment profile. Some good possibilities are nortriptyline (sold as Pamelor) and desipramine (sold as Norpramin). Often migraine can be controlled satisfactorily with very low once-a-day doses of these drugs—a level at which migraineurs report few, if any, troublesome side effects.

In a 1991 article, headache authority Dr. Seymour Diamond suggested that indeed any tricyclic antidepressant can be expected to substantially relieve migraine symptoms. According to Dr. Diamond the choice of a particular drug should hinge on two considerations—minimizing unpleasant reactions and improving any existing sleep disturbance, such as insomnia or early morning wakefulness. Some tricyclics, such as amitriptyline (Elavil) and doxepin (Sinequan or Adapin), have sedative effects and thus can bring an added benefit for sufferers who experience these sleep-related difficulties.

In addition to the traditional tricyclic family, two other categories of antidepressants are sometimes used as migraine preventives. These are the monoamine oxidase inhibitors (MAOIs), an old drug largely abandoned in migraine treatment for a time because of the complications encountered, and serotonin-uptake inhibitors (Prozac is the most popular brand), a new type of medication whose promise as a migraine preventive is only now starting to be recognized.

MAOIs are usually retained for use in severe migraineurs who are unresponsive to other medications. These drugs interfere with the production of an enzyme called monoamine oxidase, which is responsible for breaking down dietary amines in the body. Its effectiveness as a migraine preventive is well documented, but seems rather ironic in view of the fact that at least some migraineurs, that is, those falling in the dietary subgroup, are suspected of already being deficient in this particular enzyme. New, less troublesome members of this drug family have been developed and tested in the past decade, but most doctors are probably not sufficiently informed to feel comfortable prescribing them.

If you want to try one of these drugs, you most likely will need to approach a neurologist or a psychiatrist about it. Two big advantages of these drugs over the more traditional tricyclics is that the MAOIs are less likely to interfere with heart rhythms and are less drying as well. For those reasons, they sometimes are used in older patients who would not be able to tolerate the other medications. The big drawback to the MAOIs is that, in spite of recent improvements, they still require adherence to a special diet and strict avoidance of certain medications. Thus, they usually are reserved for only the most conscientious patient and one who has failed to respond to other medications. Sometimes these drugs are used together with tricyclics, a combination that seems to minimize dietary reactions.

A relatively new class of antidepressants called serotonin-uptake inhibitors has received a lot of press—some good and some bad. Although Prozac (fluoxetine) is the best known of this new drug family, close cousins are Paxil (paroxetine) and Zoloft (sertraline). Currently Prozac is used by more people than any other antidepressant, and many users testify that they are obtaining substantial relief from depression and other symptoms, including migraine, without the unpleasant side effects experienced from older antidepressants. On the other hand, a small number of users or their survivors have claimed that this drug causes either extreme anxiety or violent behavior—even going so far as to attribute murder and suicide to its use. Extensive tests and investigations by the FDA have found no support for these extreme allegations, however. Even Ralph Nader's Public Citizen Health Research Group, known for its thorough and cautious stance regarding the use of medications, recognizes the benefits of Prozac, asking merely for slightly more stringent labeling requirements. Physicians, and others familiar with the way antidepressants do their job, recognize that there is an increased risk of suicide among all severely depressed individuals when they first begin to take any antidepressant. Participating in talk therapy (counseling) along with a drug regimen seems to decrease that risk significantly. In the meantime, amid all the public furor surrounding Prozac, it is quietly proving itself an effective and desirable migraine preventive.

Some experts do note, however, that Prozac can cause as well as cure headache. In clinical trials, subjects taking this drug report experiencing headache as a side effect slightly more often than do those taking an inactive look-alike drug. In addition, hypoglycemia (low blood sugar) is a side effect of Prozac that could be important for migraineurs since that condition is known sometimes to worsen headache. Dosage seems to be critical—a fact evidently not recognized by the manufacturer Eli Lilly, who until recently made the drug in only one strength. It is now available as a liquid, allowing for easier dosage adjustment, but this form is extremely expensive. Patients who need to adjust their dose have other options, some of which are discussed later in this chapter under "Prozac: A Personal Journey."

Describing their recent study of Prozac in migraine prevention, researchers from Louisiana State University School of Medicine report that this drug achieved significant reductions in symptoms (beginning with weeks three and four of treatment) among nine migraineurs completing the trial—and without serious side effects. Some of these sufferers took the standard 20-mg dose of the drug, and others reduced their dose to half that amount during the course of the study and still were able to obtain significant relief. The researchers conclude that Prozac appears to be both safe and effective as a migraine preventive; furthermore, because the drug is designed to affect only serotonin, they cite its effectiveness as a support for the serotonin deficiency theory of migraine causality.

Still, most doctors prefer the tricyclics, which have been more widely studied and used in migraine treatment, over this newer class of drugs. Prozac is usually reserved for patients who desire to avoid the weight gain that sometimes comes with even low doses of the tricyclics. (I'd guess that most women under age 80 harbor that concern!) Some patients believe that Prozac will actually help them lose weight, a mistaken hope, according to most specialists. The only patients who might lose weight as a result of the drug, they emphasize, are those taking very high doses. And such patients might well be experiencing many unpleasant side effects, including uncomfortable anxiety and daily headaches, at the same time they are shedding a few pounds.

Another new antidepressant, trazodone, usually sold as Deseryl, also is touted as offering basically the same benefits as the older drugs, minus many of the unpleasant side effects—much in the same way that Prozac is promoted. It, too, seems to have a downside, however, with some users complaining of fatigue, anxiety, and muddled thinking. Dr. Seymour Solomon, Director of the Headache Unit at Montefiore, New York, Medical Center, suggests that this drug is useful for obese migraineurs who wish to take an antidepressant, but need to avoid gaining additional weight, a side effect often associated with the older drugs. Other sources caution against using this drug as a migraine preventive, suggesting that it is ineffective. Subjects taking Deseryl in clinical trials report headache as a frequent side effect. Dr. Sheftell points out that a byproduct of Deseryl actually causes migraine in some patients, and therefore he believes it is not the best choice for headache sufferers.

Because most of the antidepressants in current use seem to offer relief from migraine, it is tempting to think that all will function in this manner. Research suggests otherwise. At least with some of the newer drugs that have not been extensively tested or used as migraine preventives, judgment will have to be withheld until more information is available. For instance, some early tests with the antidepressant clomipramine (usually sold as Anafranil) strongly suggest that it is not an effective migraine preventive. In fact, some authorities hold that Anafranil, like Deseryl, actually worsens migraine.

Using Antidepressants

Something important to remember about using antidepressants is that they, like most other migraine preventives, do not show their full effect right away. In fact, the level of these drugs must build up in the body before they reach an effective level—a process sometimes taking up to three or four weeks. A related advantage is that, once this initial level is achieved, missing an occasional dose is usually not harmful.

Dr. Sheftell shares the following helpful information about antidepressants as well as other common preventive medications: Women with headaches that either worsen or occur only in association with their menstrual period (or the estrogen dip around that time) may find relief by taking these drugs only during that vulnerable phase, or by taking a low dose of the medications all month and then increasing it before the expected event.

Of course, there are real and serious contraindications to the use of antidepressants, as well as potentially adverse side effects associated with the drugs. One potentially troublesome side effect from antidepressants, sometimes even at low doses, stems from the tendency of these drugs to lower blood sugar levels. These lower levels in turn may trigger headaches unless special care is taken. (*See* Chapter 4 for more information on scheduling food intake to minimize blood sugar problems.) Another downside to these drugs is their tendency to make patients more susceptible to sunburn, a fact often not mentioned by doctors but with a potential for painful and even dangerous consequences. Some drug manuals warn that these drugs can contribute to gum disease in predisposed people, a side effect that both my friend and I seem to have experienced from Prozac. Good dental hygiene and frequent exams are recommended.

Other Preventives

Methysergide Maleate

Usually sold as Sansert, this drug is the only one other than propranolol (Inderal) and cousin beta blocker timolol (Blocadren) that is recognized by the FDA specifically as an effective migraine preventive. Yet, potential side effects are so dangerous that many physicians are reluctant to prescribe it. Others, expert in the field, believe that the drug is safe and effective as long as it is used continuously for no more than 4–6 months. They then require a brief "vacation" from the medication in order to avoid possible scar tissue formation or development of a serious blood disorder. Sansert causes some other unpleasant side effects, which even apart from the scary ones, probably would make it a drug of last resort, reserved for difficult cases. These include depression, fluid retention, muscle cramps, and abdominal discomfort.

NSAIDs

Although these nonsteroidal anti-inflammatory drugs are considered effective migraine preventives as well as abortives, gastrointestinal symptoms frequently caused by their *regular daily use* may make them unwise for many sufferers. On the other hand, for people in whom changes in blood pressure and cardiac conduction are undesirable and for whom gastrointestinal irritation does not present a serious risk, these drugs may be a better choice than the beta or calcium blockers. The NSAIDs do not directly alter blood vessel tone as do both the blocker families, but long-term daily use of these drugs may cause or worsen kidney problems; this situation can be monitored through simple blood tests.

A regimen of twice daily administration of 550 mg of either naproxen sodium (Anaprox or Aleve) or naproxen (Naprosyn) is sometimes recommended as one that achieves good control with few side effects. Several other prescription NSAIDs are often recommended for migraine as well. Sufferers are also finding the nonprescription drug ibuprofen helpful. Indeed, patient response to this drug family seems to be quite individualized. Some experts suggest that simple trial and error may be the only way for a sufferer to find the best medication.

Even if a sufferer is afraid to risk the possible gastrointestinal consequences of daily NSAID use, these drugs can be a helpful addition to other preventives or can serve as occasional preventives in their own right—roles that frequently seem to be overlooked by both migraineur and doctor. Examples of such use include taking these drugs for approximately one week out of each menstrual cycle in women who suffer from premenstrual or menstrual headache, or taking them before a flight to prevent symptoms caused by rapidly changing air pressure in airline cabins.

Aspirin

Some migraineurs take regular daily doses of aspirin as part of a self-directed prevention program. Experts question the wisdom of such long-term use, cautioning that it actually may interfere with the body's natural pain fighting mechanism, thereby worsening the headache disorder. However, now that recent studies have demonstrated the value of aspirin in helping to prevent both stroke and heart attack, very low daily doses seem to make sense as part of a migraine prevention program as well.

Many authorities believe that when blood platelets aggregate or stick together, they tend to dump their serotonin content; this serotonin dumping, in turn, may be an early event in the snowball reaction leading to a migraine attack. Indeed, as was mentioned earlier, the Physicians' Health Study specifically showed that taking 325 mg of aspirin every other day was associated with a 20% reduction in migraine frequency. British authority Dr. Edda Hanington advises that this anticlumping effect can be achieved most effectively with very low daily doses, just 50 mg—an amount equivalent to only slightly more than one half a children's (baby) aspirin. Some researchers recommend even smaller amounts.

I was reluctant to try the low-dose aspirin because regular pain-killing doses invariably gave me heartburn. After an enteric (coated to dissolve in the intestine rather than the stomach) 81 mg tablet became available, however, I decided to add this to my regimen. (Such a product is made by both Bayer and Halfprin.) I took this low-dose tablet four days a week and found that it further raised my migraine threshold. In fact for the first time in over a dozen years, I was able to fly without getting a headache. After a couple of weeks on the coated aspirin, I was dismayed to note the beginning of abdominal discomfort a few hours after swallowing my dose. I certainly did not want to give up the benefits, but the abdominal pain was both distressing and somewhat worrisome. Fortunately I found myself able to tolerate taking three quarters of a chewable baby aspirin on a daily basis. Even though the enteric product is advertised as being easier on the digestive tract, that certainly was not my experience. As an added bonus: the baby aspirin is both less expensive and easier to remember taking (a daily routine becomes automatic) than the stronger special variety I took only every other day.

Several of my friends have tried this simple preventive measure and report improvement from it as well.

Just remember that these very low doses are probably far better for migraine prevention than higher amounts, although the best exact dose for this purpose has not yet been established by research. If you decide to try this simple, inexpensive, and usually safe strategy, discuss it with your doctor first. Be alert that too much aspirin can result in easy bruising and even an increased risk of a certain type of stroke. Many physicians recommend that even low-dose aspirin be stopped two weeks prior to *any* surgical/dental procedures. And to be on the safe side, even low doses should be taken with food or milk (or, for further stomach protection, dissolved and drunk in the liquid).

Fish Oil Supplements

Some preliminary evidence suggests that Omega Three fish oil supplements may decrease migraine incidence. Such a benefit is thought to result from the oil's interference with platelet clumping in the blood, just as is the case with aspirin.

The long-term safety of this product has not yet been demonstrated, however, and its purity and potency are poorly regulated. A more immediate difficulty for migraineurs is the tendency of these oils to lower blood sugar levels and thus lead to an even greater number of headaches. (Indeed I had exactly that experience when I tried this product a few years ago, although I did not understand the reason until I was researching the matter later.) Migraineurs should consult their personal physicians before using even nonprescription products.

Feverfew

An herbal remedy, long used in Europe to combat headache and other maladies, this over-the-counter product has demonstrated significant ability to reduce migraine incidence in controlled trials. Here again, however, at least in this country, purity and potency of herbal products are very poorly regulated, making appropriate dosage maintenance impossible, and long-term safety has not been shown. In fact, a serious blood disorder may result from prolonged use of this agent. Consult your doctor if you are thinking of using this as a migraine preventive.

Antihistamines

Cyproheptadine (sold as Periactin, a prescription medication), although technically an antihistamine, also changes the serotonin system and has shown impressive ability to prevent migraine attacks. Unfortunately, unpleasant side effects—including dry mouth, sleepiness, and a tendency for increased appetite and weight gain—make it unattractive for long-term use. However, it seems to be one of those agents, like the NSAIDs, that can be used successfully as an occasional preventive. Drs. Rapoport and Sheftell recommend its use to combat both menstrual migraine and attacks experienced when withdrawing from oral contraceptives.

I believe that another antihistamine, specifically chlorpheniramine (sold as Chlor-Trimeton, or generic versions thereof, and available in convenient timed-release forms) can be used in much the same way—as an occasional preventive. No controlled studies verify the effectiveness of this drug in migraine treatment, but I know several migraineurs who find it extremely helpful. Apparently most antihistamines have at least some effect on neurotransmitter systems as well as on histamine, and thus seem to stabilize blood vessels.

Unfortunately, any of these drugs that is strong enough to be of significant help in migraine control is drying (constipation is a common side effect) and is apt to cause drowsiness as well. The newer, gentler antihistamines, like Seldane, are unlikely to be much help for any except the mildest migraine symptoms. I have found, however, that by taking only half the recommended dose of generic chlorpheniramine, I can minimize side effects while still getting relief. I take this drug prior to both dust and pollen exposure (some of my triggers) as well as before airline trips, and between the time I have eaten an offending food and the time I expect a reaction. If you try this last maneuver, you'll need to arrange the timing to allow for your own biological clock; the drug must be taken before symptoms appear. Prior to starting Prozac, my current preventative, I was actually able to stave off severe attacks by taking this drug around the clock, on a daily basis, for months at a time. The only reason I discontinued it was because of severe constipation. This drug's other major downside was its failure to improve my low moods and lagging energy level.

Newer Medications

Research trials continue to explore other drugs for possible use as migraine preventives. Drugs currently being evaluated are valproic acid (sold as Depakote, Myproic Acid, and other brand names), an antiseizure drug that many believe is showing great promise as a migraine treatment, as well as the blood pressure medications captopril (Capoten) and enalapril (Vasotec).

Biofeedback: Natural Chemical Warfare

Biofeedback, a medically directed and mechanically monitored program of relaxation training, is an impressive tool for both avoiding and relieving migraine. Experts believe it works by stimulating production of the body's natural vasodilating and pain-relieving chemicals, thus counteracting the troublesome noradrenaline produced in stressful situations. Not surprisingly, this technique seems to work much better in fighting stress-triggered headaches than those triggered by dietary or hormonal factors, although it sometimes may help the latter as well. Your physician can refer you to a special treatment center where a team of trained medical professionals will instruct you in relaxation skills, measure your progress, and give you "feedback" by means of painless sensors that are attached to your forehead or finger to detect blood flow.

As part of the training, you will be asked to practice new skills at home for about 20 minutes a day, perhaps with the help of audio tapes. You may be given a finger monitor to use during these at-home practice sessions. On average, about ten in-office visits are required to teach relaxation skills in this way. Experts generally advise that migraineurs must actually use biofeedback daily for about six weeks before judging its effectiveness. They also warn that certain medications, including daily analgesics, tranquilizers, and even beta blockers, interfere with learning biofeedback and other relaxation skills and tend to negate their potential benefits. Cost for the training no doubt varies according to area and among practitioners—one clinic in the MidAtlantic region charges $1000 for the basic training—and, as often as not, the training program will not be covered by medical insurance.

Migraineurs probably have not taken full advantage of the help this tool can offer—possibly because it does require a substantial investment of time, effort, and sometimes personal money as well. Lack of understanding about what is involved also may cause some of us to hesitate seeking this effective treatment. Chapter 4 of the book *Headache Relief* (Rapoport and Sheftell, 1991) does an excellent job of describing exactly what biofeedback training entails. This treatment is especially valuable during pregnancy or nursing, when most drugs are not considered safe, and for children or others whose pain syndromes are not firmly entrenched.

Combination Treatments: Hope and Fear

In addition to the treatment already mentioned in which two types of antidepressants, a tricyclic and an MAOI, are used together in previously nonresponsive patients, there is another popular combination treatment involving the use of a tricyclic antidepressant with propranolol (Inderal). Dr. N. T. Mathew, Director of the Houston Headache Clinic, describes an interesting study conducted at his clinic in which these two drugs were combined with biofeedback for use with a large group of mixed headache patients. The patients receiving all three treatments reported significantly greater relief than comparable groups receiving any one of them alone, and there were no adverse interactions among the three. Dr. Mathew also cites the results of another study in which propranolol (Inderal) and amitriptyline (Elavil) were used together with equally good results in relieving otherwise unresponsive headache symptoms.

The most effective treatment of any tested under controlled conditions appears to be a combination of diet, beta blocker, biofeedback, and behavioral therapy, including both individual and family counseling. In an impressive study of this holistic approach, also conducted at the Houston Headache Clinic under the auspices of Dr. Mathew, 76% of sufferers showed a significant reduction in headache frequency and severity, an improvement that continued during a three-year followup period.

I have serious concerns about the way some of these combination drug treatments are commonly used, however. The usual procedure is to put a patient on a beta blocker for a trial period; if improvement is not satisfactory, the doctor often then adds an antidepressant to her regimen. Less often is a trial given to the antidepressant alone to see whether response to that drug is adequate. This popular combination approach increases the likelihood that a patient will be overmedicated, risking unpleasant and possibly dangerous side effects. A better method, in my opinion, would be to try each drug alone before considering combining them.

Prozac: A Personal Journey

I was in my late thirties when my attacks struck with a vengeance. In retrospect, I realize that I had experienced mild migraine symptoms as an adolescent, but at that time had been totally unaware of the nature of my malady. In fact, even after my symptoms became severe, several years passed before I was able to obtain a correct diagnosis—let alone any medical relief. That early help, such as it was, came in the form of my reluctant use of ergotamine and cafergot—unhappy experiences I have already described earlier in this chapter.

Fortunately during much of that first migraine decade, I was able to control my symptoms through a holistic lifestyle regimen—that is by attending to all the factors outlined in earlier chapters, including maintaining regular eating and sleeping schedules; eliminating caffeine and alcohol, and restricting or avoiding offending foods; implementing a regular aerobic exercise program; and learning new ways to deal with stress. I felt more comfortable using these measures rather than resorting to daily medication—largely because of some early life experiences that resulted in a cautious, if not actually fearful, attitude toward medical treatment. My mother had suffered permanent brain damage from the electro-convulsive shock treatments she received for depression when I was ten years old—an experience that left me extremely hesitant to consider any regular use of medication. As my symptoms became more severe, of course, maintaining that cautious stance became increasingly painful. My research into preventive medication began in earnest at that point.

I did not believe I was an appropriate candidate for beta blockers both because of tendencies toward bronchial allergies and the relatively poor blood flow in my hands and feet. My reading indicated that long-term side effects might be a legitimate concern with the betas as well. I was especially wary of increased stroke risk since I already faced a strong family history of early strokes. Calcium channel blockers seemed less effective and could certainly have unpleasant side effects as well.

Antidepressants, on the other hand, appealed to my logical nature because their action in relieving migraines is better understood and apparently more straightforward than that of the other popular drug families. It is well understood that antidepressants act directly on neurotransmitter systems in the brain, the very chemicals implicated in causing migraine. A definite bonus for me in choosing an antidepressant for migraine control was the likelihood that it would also relieve some relatively low-level symptoms of depression from which I had suffered on and off all my life. These seemed to be worse as I approached menopause, perhaps because of hormonal changes; but the bouts certainly had not been helped by a decade of battling severe pain.

My interest in antidepressants heightened when I heard about Prozac, an innovative drug reportedly free of some of the troublesome side effects associated with the earlier medications—namely dry mouth, constipation, weight gain, and interference with normal heart rhythms. I was pleased to discover that preliminary research confirmed its effectiveness as a migraine preventive, and after overcoming an initial reluctance, based on a fear of what other people might think, I decided to consult a psychiatrist, the specialist with the greatest expertise in prescribing antidepressants. The doctor I chose had the reputation for being extremely knowledgeable, but yet quite cautious, in his use of drugs. If he agreed with my request for Prozac, I knew I would feel confident trying it.

After a lengthy discussion and evaluation, the psychiatrist started me on the standard Prozac dose, a daily 20-mg capsule, to be taken in the morning with food. Over the course of the next few months, I was to see a great improvement in both my low-level depression and my excruciating migraine symptoms. I also noted a welcome increase in my energy level—a frequent result of antidepressants. Initially I experienced some irritating side effects, for which the doctor had prepared me, namely bizarre dreams and morning anxiety, perhaps best described as "coffee nerves."

The morning anxiety passed after the first week, and although the odd dreams persisted to some extent, they seemed a small price indeed for the improvement in the quality of my life that the medication had brought. My severe attacks stopped, and most of the mild migraines I did experience responded very well to over-the-counter pain relievers.

Several months into the treatment, however, I began to experience some more troublesome symptoms—increased anxiety, especially shortly before meals and sometimes including rather severe disorientation—and almost daily headaches that seemed to be stress related. When my reading led to the realization that such symptoms might result from too much Prozac, I returned to my doctor for a dosage adjustment. Like Goldilocks, I had to experiment—first too hot, then too cold! Half a capsule apparently was not enough—I experienced breakthrough episodes of both depression and migraines with that level; two-thirds of a capsule proved just right: no depression, few migraine symptoms, and few troublesome side effects. Those of you severe sufferers who have experienced similar success in using medication will be able to understand the relief I felt.

After I began hormone supplementation, I was successfully able to reduce my daily Prozac intake to one-half capsule. The only downside of using the two agents together, for me at least, is that they seem to have adversely affected my blood sugar so that I must be especially careful about eating on time. Now that I have worked out a satisfactory level of the medication, the psychiatrist has discharged me, turning the supervision of my Prozac over to my family practitioner. As the medical community gains more experience in using this drug in general, and for migraine prevention in particular, family practitioners probably will feel comfortable prescribing it, as indeed many of them now do with the older antidepressants.

Because Prozac initially was available in only one strength, I had to be somewhat creative about accomplishing the required dose reductions. To make the two-thirds capsule, I had to dump out the contents of two capsules and repackage them in three empty gelcaps purchased from my pharmacy; the half dose was simpler—I simply sliced each capsule into two approximately equal portions with a sharp single-edged razor blade and then inserted each half into one of the gelcaps. Another option suggested by my doctor was to empty the contents of a capsule in a measured amount of juice, drinking an appropriate portion and saving the rest for another day.

Fortunately Prozac is now available in both a liquid and a newer 10 mg capsule, making dose adjustments much easier. If you try dose reductions with it or any other medication, please do so only with the consent of your doctor. And be aware that Prozac is a mucous-membrane irritant that should be kept away from the eyes and other sensitive tissue. For the same reason, this drug should be taken with food or milk in order to avoid heartburn.

Finding the Prozac dose that was right for me proved to be far more challenging than I ever would have guessed. This experience alerted me to the importance of joint doctor–patient cooperation in identifying the correct level of any migraine preventive. Much of my reading has highlighted the importance of this matter. Not only physicians but we migraineurs as well have been somewhat lax about this important consideration. After all, a magic pill should work magically—without a great deal of effort on our parts! On the contrary, I found that fine tuning my Prozac dose took months of frustrating, painful experimentation, with assistance from an understanding physician who was willing to give me some leeway.

Realistic Treatment Expectations: Utopia Revisited

What can we realistically expect from a migraine preventive? Most experts agree that it is unreasonable to think any preventive medication will eliminate severe migraine symptoms completely and for all time. Even propranolol (Inderal), which is judged by many to be the most effective preventive, reduces symptoms by no more than 50%. Some researchers question even that relatively optimistic claim; using a different statistical method to analyze data from the clinical trials of the drug, they interpret it to mean only a 25% improvement.

Migraine patients have noticed, as well, that sometimes preventive medication that works well initially loses its effectiveness over time. A study at the Houston Headache Center found that 16% of patients taking a beta blocker experienced a failure in effectiveness after several years on that medication; 12% of those taking methysergide (Sansert) had a similar failure.

Sufferers who begin preventive medication with the expectation of banishing symptoms are almost certainly doomed to disappointment. Most sufferers can, however, with persistent effort and help from a knowledgeable physician, eventually find substantial relief. In order to accomplish this challenging "balancing act"—maximizing relief while keeping unpleasant side effects at a minimum—many of us will need to begin or continue an accompanying holistic lifestyle regimen in addition to our medical treatment. With an effective combination of the two types of treatment, doses of pain-relieving drugs usually can be reduced to a manageable level, even by the severe sufferer. Periodic reevaluations and sometimes complete changes may be indicated.

On a personal level, to summarize how my preventive medication has affected me, I would say that it has reset my migraine threshold, so that greater trigger exposure must now occur to provoke an attack, and pain-relieving medication that was once totally ineffective is now surprisingly successful in eliminating 90% of symptoms. My energy level is noticeably higher. In short, Prozac has radically changed my life. Hormone supplements, low-dose aspirin, and magnesium supplements have reduced my headaches still further and have made me much more comfortable.

Some practitioners advise discontinuing preventive medication after about six months of good control in order to see whether or not attacks have stopped permanently. If they return, then medication can be started again. (When daily preventive medication is discontinued, symptoms frequently do not reappear for as long as two months or more.) The severe sufferer may object to this strategy because most preventive agents must build up to a certain level in the body before becoming fully effective, perhaps leaving the migraineur vulnerable for a time. On the other hand, if preventives are continued indefinitely, then a sufferer may not realize it when a threshold is somehow reset and the migraines cease, making daily medication unnecessary. Another of the many quandaries to be faced when living with migraine!

One sensible approach is to wean oneself gradually from the daily preventive while remaining on guard for a possible return of symptoms. In my own case, after I began taking Prozac, I increased my magnesium supplements and started both hormone replacement therapy and a low-dose aspirin regimen. Therefore I considered it wise to reevaluate my situation by attempting to reduce my Prozac dose. Unfortunately I did not fare well when such an attempt was made. My old symptoms began to recur, and I quickly returned to previous levels, facing the prospect of long-term Prozac use. I consider myself lucky that the medication continues to work well for me.

The Pendulum Swings: *Undertreatment*

For decades, before the development of effective preventive medications, various narcotics commonly were prescribed for migraine, and it was not unusual for sufferers to become addicted to those drugs. Later, troublesome or even serious problems arose in the form of habituation and rebound headache, not only from ergot but from many of the barbiturates taken to control pain as well. To further complicate the situation, nonmigraine sufferers sometimes faked headache pain in order to persuade doctors to prescribe addictive drugs. Because of all these difficulties, and perhaps also because physicians themselves are not always well versed in current options, some of today's doctors seem overly reluctant to prescribe appropriate preventive and/or abortive medications, and some medical insurance carriers no longer pay for emergency room treatment of migraine.

Considering this situation from the migraineur's point of view, many of us continue to suffer needlessly because of *our own* attitudes. We may harbor fears from past experiences—either our own or those of our acquaintances—or simply because we, too, lack information about available choices. A stoic reluctance to seek help seems especially common among older sufferers and among those who have experienced migraine most or all of their lives. The latter group appears particularly resigned to their pain as a natural and inevitable part of their personal lot in life. Undoubtedly, some of these reluctant patients have received critical messages from doctors or others at some time, implying that they are neurotic complainers or that their headaches are psychological in origin. As I have already admitted, I was stubbornly reluctant to seek help as well; but now that I have obtained it, I deeply regret waiting so long to ask.

The Big Picture: *Medical Treatments*

If you are ready to begin the process of trying to find effective medical treatment, rereading Chapter 1 may be of value; it provides suggestions about how to identify a helpful physician and then to work with that doctor to achieve the best possible approach.

Also remember to complete Appendix G to clarify whether or not a preventive medication is appropriate for you. And, above all, please don't forget the frequent necessity for fine tuning both choice and dose of drugs. In summary, keep the following points in mind as you consider or use migraine medication:

1. There is no medical *cure* for migraine, but there are treatments that will reduce symptoms significantly.
2. Mastering biofeedback is probably worthwhile, especially if stress is a primary trigger and you are reluctant to learn relaxation skills on your own.
3. Unless a particular treatment improves overall well-being, then that treatment is a failure.
4. To minimize unwanted side effects, keep dosage low by starting or continuing a holistic lifestyle regimen.
5. The choice of a particular drug(s) is a personal matter, based on coexisting conditions, individual preference, and lifestyle. Often some side effects must be tolerated; only you can decide whether or not they are worthwhile.
6. Identifying the right dosage is just as important, at least in many cases, as selecting the most helpful medication.
7. In general, research supports the following conclusions about particular treatments, although considerable variation exists because of factors outlined in # 5 above:
   a. To interrupt a severe attack at home, Imitrex appears to offer a breakthrough in effective treatment. Ergot continues to help many people,

and the NSAIDs, although less potent still offer a favorable benefit/
risk ratio.

b. In a medical setting, Reglan probably is safe and effective for most
patients. It is important to observe dosage restrictions with all
migraine abortive agents.

c. Daily pain relievers should be avoided because they tend to interfere
with the natural pain system and probably worsen headache in the
long run.

d. Low-dose aspirin may be worth a trial for many patients as a preventive strategy.

e. Among other preventives, antidepressants seem to offer the best treatment profile, especially when low doses provide effective control.
Specifically favorable are Pamelor, Norpramin, and Prozac. Among
the beta blockers, Tenormin, in moderate doses, probably offers the
most favorable profile. Many people find relief with the calcium channel blocker Calan; and Cardizem looks promising.

f. It is best to avoid narcotics and barbiturates as pain relievers or sedatives; Tylenol is relatively ineffective.

g. As occasional preventives, both NSAIDs and Periactin may be
helpful.

Balance to Be Achieved

To find the medication(s) that will relieve symptoms most effectively,
with the fewest unpleasant or dangerous short and long-term side effects.

Chapter 11

Healing the Scars

Getting Better After Your Headaches Do

Would a Benign Illness Leave Scars?

From a technical, medical point of view, migraine is commonly called a "benign" disorder, meaning that it is not life-threatening. Somehow, although intellectually understanding the basic intent of that label, I have always found it rather insensitive. It's very difficult for anyone who has experienced the excruciating pain and disability of severe migraine even to think of that experience in the same breath as the word "benign." I guess, at least emotionally, that designation represents for me the ultimate oxymoron.

The medical profession now does recognize, and belatedly has begun to address, some of the physical scars of migraine. Dr. J. N. Blau, British migraine expert, at least acknowledges that pain can continue for days or even weeks after a severe attack. Blau calls that period the "postdrome," which he likens to the symptoms of a hangover. Forty-seven out of 50 sufferers interviewed by Blau in 1982 reported experiencing such an aftermath to their attacks.

My personal postdrome at times has persisted for several weeks, marked by minor hearing loss, an unpleasant feeling of head fullness, occasional throbbing, and periodic spells of weakness and lightheadedness; all of these symptoms were worse when I was reclining, thus requiring that I sleep in an uncomfortable, propped-up position. Certainly not life-threatening, but hardly my idea of fun either.

Recent research has confirmed a long-harbored suspicion linking migraine to a somewhat increased risk of stroke, rendering the headache disorder less than benign according to anyone's perspective.

However, the most disabling scars left behind by severe chronic migraine are probably psychological rather than physical. This disorder is so disruptive to a person's normal lifestyle that it almost inevitably wreaks havoc, havoc that is felt not only within the individual sufferer, but within the context of close relationships as well. (Reviewing the section on stress in Chapter 4 may be helpful in dealing with some of these problems.)

Migraine and Depression: *The Chicken and the Egg*

Living with migraine is a challenge at best. At worst it leaves us feeling as if our lives are spinning out of control. Fighting this powerful disorder year after year can be exhausting and eventually downright depressing. In fact, as some psychologists point out, it is precisely when we feel as if we're losing control, when the headache process has taken over our position in the driver's seat, that depression is apt to catch us in its vise. Ironically, depression can become a rather familiar, even comfortable, rut, so don't be surprised if, after you get a handle on your migraines, it takes you a significant period of time, perhaps even several months, to climb out of that rut.

Recovery can be complicated by the gradual onset of the depression. Sometimes the affected individual is not even aware that the condition is developing. After all, when you're busy fighting migraine, there's not much time or energy to devote to anything else. Additionally, in general, an individual tends to be a poor judge of her own moods. It might be helpful to ask your significant other and good friends whether they have noticed any changes in your mood or attitude over the months or years you've been experiencing migraines. Are you more irritable, more negative, less patient, or even significantly less daring than you were before the worsening of your migraine condition? Talking with intimates about these matters can be enlightening.

The bottom line in this situation seems to be identifying which came first in your life, the depression or the migraines. Certainly, as I have indicated, chronic severe migraines can contribute to a depressed mood; but on the other hand, as researchers tell us, anxiety and depression actually precede headache in 20–40% of migraineurs. Experts believe that many migraineurs who experience depression probably suffer from an inherited form of that illness, that is, an inborn biochemically induced condition somehow linked to their migraine predisposition. It is not expected, then, that these individuals will be able to pull themselves out of depression by their bootstraps. They may benefit greatly from an antidepressant medication as treatment for both their headaches and their depressed mood.

If, after about six months of persistent self-help, you continue to feel down much of the time, noting a lack of enjoyment in everyday experiences, then it might be appropriate to seek a professional counselor, social worker, or psychologist to guide you in your psychological recovery. Other possible symptoms of depression include hopelessness about the future, frequent crying, thoughts or plans of suicide, unusual fatigue, trouble concentrating, difficulty in falling asleep or sleeping normally through the night, a large weight loss or gain, and a decrease in sexual interest and/or response. (For a reminder about the relationship between depression and migraine, as well as more detailed information on the use of antidepressant medication in migraine treatment, you may want to reread Chapters 8 and 10.)

Psychiatrists are the medical specialists with the greatest expertise in prescribing antidepressant medications. In fact in today's medical community, contrary to popular opinion, the chief function of that specialty is the dispensation and management of drugs, rather than psychoanalysis in the classical tradition. Today, other medical professionals usually conduct any needed counseling. In spite of the stigma still attached to seeing a psychiatrist, I decided to consult such a physician when I became interested in trying a preventive regimen with the controversial drug Prozac. I found that doctor quite skilled in supervising such treatment and have never regretted entrusting my care to him.

Smelling the Roses

Preliminary research suggests that increasing pleasurable and rewarding activities can bring health benefits, including strengthening both the immune system and the body's natural pain-fighting mechanisms. Much has been written about this mind–body connection since it was discussed by Dr. William Glasser in his *Positive Addiction* (1976) and by Norman Cousins in his *Anatomy of an Illness* (1979). Indeed I am indebted to both Glasser and Cousins for much of my holistic philosophy. Because of the wide treatment of this philosophy in popular literature, my present consideration of it will be very brief.

Both the immune and pain-fighting systems (thought to benefit from an increase in pleasurable activity) are regarded by many as deficient in migraineurs. Increasing pleasurable activity, then, makes sense for us in at least two different ways. It may help correct biological deficiencies that contribute to our disorder; at the same time such activities likely will help us to counteract the doldrums arising from our frustrating struggle and to regain a more positive outlook on life. Let's get to "play" then.

Fun Is Where You Find It

Obviously the definition of a pleasurable or rewarding activity varies tremendously from one person to another. My counseling clients who have explored this same topic often list the following activities as ones that bring them pleasure:

1. Music—playing an instrument, listening at home, or attending concerts
2. Handwork or mechanical hobbies—sewing, building models, or refinishing furniture, for example
3. Gardening—inside or out
4. Sports activities—watching or playing; individual or team
5. Sexual encounters—consistent with your personal code of morality; and most beneficial, I would think, within the context of a loving relationship

The common element among these activities is their ability to cause participants to lose themselves in the process; by means of such pursuits, we are able, for a time, to escape our problems, our worries, and even, if we are lucky, our very selves. Such escape is usually psychologically healthful, as long as it's not done to excess. In a way, this type of escape takes the place of what many people seek through alcohol and other drugs, thus giving rise to Glasser's use of the phrase "positive addiction."

Many psychologists encourage increased interaction with supportive friends and pets as one important means of increasing pleasure in our lives. Starting a headache support group in your own community would be one way to arrange for ongoing empathetic contacts as well as a resource center. The American Council for Headache Education (ACHE) offers material for organizing such groups. (*See* Chapter 1 for ACHE's address.)

Norman Cousins popularized the notion of courting laughter—feeling comfortable laughing at ourselves, learning and sharing puns and jokes, and increasing the time we spend listening to or watching our favorite comics. When I was at my lowest point and house-bound much of the time, I started a humor network—exchanging jokes (political satire is my favorite) with friends by phone and letter.

Paradoxical as it may seem, many of us have discovered that one sure way to increase our pleasure is by helping others. Opportunities for this kind of self-fulfillment are ever present. Think of the Red Cross blood drives, adult literacy and school tutoring programs, nursing home and hospital volunteer requirements, food bank and animal shelter needs, winterizing or building-repair efforts, local soup kitchen projects, Big Brother/Big Sister activities, and Scouting programs, just to name a few. If you are new to a community, your local United Way, Salvation Army, or city or county social services agency probably can provide some suggestions for meaningful volunteer work.

If you tend to be a little shy or for any reason prefer to avoid one-on-one contact, please realize that you can help others in relatively impersonal ways and still feel a strong sense of personal satisfaction. Your time and effort spent chopping vegetables in a soup kitchen or providing clerical assistance in a hospital undoubtedly would be appreciated by others and psychologically healthful for you as well. I get a kick out of both types of activity. For example, giving blood (the impersonal) and tutoring children (the personal), are two of my own favorites.

If you have trouble identifying potentially pleasurable activities, try thinking back to your childhood. You might still enjoy flying a kite, putting on a pair of skates, visiting a zoo, or going on a picnic. Recently I got a front-porch swing because I loved swinging as a kid; and I still find it relaxing. I've planted a Japanese maple tree in my front yard in view of the swing to increase my enjoyment. I'm looking forward to observing the colorful seasonal changes for which this particular tree is noted.

But if you're not turned on by the prospect of rediscovering childhood pleasures, take the opposite tack: What do you look forward to doing in your golden years? Always wanted to play bridge or square dance? Why not join a group and start now? Community colleges and city recreation departments frequently offer instruction in an impressive variety of fare. Pick up your phone, order their catalogs, and you'll have a wide array of pleasurable activities from which to choose. I'd long wanted to know more about my ancestors, and so I have started to trace my family tree. In addition to using records available through my public library and the nearby Latter Day Saints' facility, I have scheduled several family vacations around visits to ancestral homes—meeting long-lost cousins and visiting other points of interest in the process.

Even if you start small, do something pleasurable. Lounging in a luxurious bubble bath or just loafing on the front stoop on the first warm day of spring is a great beginning for someone whose life has been preoccupied with surviving headache pain. Even if you have to force yourself, because you feel too down to possibly enjoy anything, pick just one rose and smell it each day.

Sometimes identifying a pleasurable activity is no problem, but fitting it into your busy life may be a challenge. If you spend most of your waking hours making a long commute and working at a job you hate, then obviously your rose-smelling time will be extremely limited. Ever considered consulting a career counselor? Community colleges may be willing to assist you. Or if changing jobs is out of the question, then simply joining a carpool or riding public transportation could possibly free up time for you to begin some reading, writing, or other creative activity. Use your imagination. Likewise, if you're the parent of preschool children and have few available baby sitters, you may well have difficulty freeing up the time for enjoyable activities. Could you join a babysitting co-op or perhaps even organize one, possibly in your neighborhood or through your church or synagogue? If you are really serious about reclaiming your life from migraine and accompanying depression, then smelling the roses needs to become a priority. And it's up to you to make it one.

On The Way To A New Life: Overcoming Bad Habits

Some tendencies I observed in myself during the period when I was suffering from severe attacks included irritability toward intimates and a reluctance to commit to activities that I had previously found rewarding. I suspect I'm not alone in exhibiting those two behavior patterns. My irritability was not confined just to the time of the actual attack; had that been the case, perhaps it would have been better understood and accepted. Rather, because the headaches were so painful and unpredictable, they colored my moods most of the time. The resulting grumpiness became habitual and left some deep scars in my relationships. Neither the habit itself nor the scars it created disappeared with the headaches. Taking Prozac, my antidepressant medication, and working with a family counselor were helpful to me in minimizing both the habit and the scars.

My reluctance toward involvement was, I believe, a logical reaction to the severe and unpredictable nature of my attacks. In my premigraine days I had been a highly motivated and rather impetuous person, eager to jump with both feet into whatever cause I felt strongly about. That all changed with the advent of migraines. Because I was too responsible to commit to something with which I might not be able to follow through, for several years I simply stopped committing. And since most of my friendships had grown out of shared activities, during that period of incapacity I formed few new relationships.

That situation did not automatically reverse itself with the improvement of my attacks either. Turning it around called for active thinking and planning on my part. I pushed myself to start a new job, and after regaining some of my self-confidence, I found the courage to apply for admission to obtain an additional graduate degree. At about the same time, I completed in-depth research on the subject of migraines, acquired a computer, developed basic word-processing skills, and began to write this book.

I feel as if my migraine scars are healing and that my life, after more than a decade of disruption, is finally back on track. I wish the same success for you.

APPENDIX A

Sample Headache–Diary Format

Date:

Day of Menstrual Cycle:

Description of Attack:

Symptoms   Time of Onset   Severity*

Medication:

Type   Time Taken   Response*

Main Activities of the Day/Changes in Sleep or Exercise Schedule:

*Rate severity and response on a scale from one to three: e.g., mild, distressing, or disabling for severity; good, fair, or poor for response.

Suspected Triggers:

Foods Eaten in Previous 36 Hours:

Breakfast   Lunch   Dinner   Snacks

Previous Day (to account for other 12 hrs).

APPENDIX B

Minimizing Migraine

A Self-Evaluation

As Chapter 3 explains, it is not unusual for people of all ages to "lose" or "gain" migraine or to experience either gradual or sudden changes in the severity of migraine symptoms—for the better or worse. Many triggers and threshold-setters with which we come into contact in the course of our everyday lives can affect our migraine symptoms without our even being aware of the connection. The list below is not all-inclusive, but it does outline many common experiences that sometimes affect migraine. If you have noticed changes in your symptoms, either recently or in the past, read through this self-evaluation and see whether or not you can relate those changes to any of the experiences listed. This is simply a guide to help you organize your thoughts on the matter. Obviously, there are no right or wrong answers, and no one else need see the sheet unless you wish to share it. Just read through it and make any appropriate notes for yourself. (Extra space is provided after each main category for brief notes.) Then, *after* you finish reading the book, go back through this guide again to see if you can think of other experiences that might have had an impact on migraine symptoms. Chapters that deal with the subject matter of each category are noted in parenthesis for your convenience. Remember, KNOWLEDGE IS POWER!

1. *Changes in Medical Conditions/Treatments* (Chapters 8 and 9)

    A. Began/Changed Blood Pressure Treatment (hypertension)
       Reserpine preparation
       Beta or calcium channel blocker
       Diuretic
       Other
    B. Began/Changed Treatment for Heart Disease
       Nitroglycerine preparation
       Beta or calcium channel blocker
       Other

   C. Diagnosis and/or Treatment for Mood Disorder (depression/anxiety)
      Antidepressant
      Tranquilizer
      Other
   D. Began/Changed treatment for Thyroid Condition
      Hypothyroidism
      Hyperthyroidism
   E. Blood Sugar Disorders Diagnosed/Treated
      Diabetes
      Low Blood Sugar
   F. Allergies/Sinus Conditions/Asthma Diagnosed/Treated
      Decongestants (especially long-lasting nasal sprays)
      Theophylline preparations (or other xanthine derivatives)
      Ephedrine or epinephrine bronchodilators
      Other sympathomimetics (*see* Chapter 9)
   G. Dental Anesthetics
   H. Surgical Anesthetics, general or local
    I. Other Changes in Medical Conditions/Treatments

2. *Recent Hormone Changes* (chiefly for females) (Chapter 7)

   A. Puberty
   B. Pregnancy
   C. Childbirth
   D. Birth Control Pill Began/Changed
   E. Approaching or Entering Menopause (Hormone changes start *about* ten years before periods cease)
   F. Hysterectomy
   G. Hormone Replacement Therapy Began/Changed

3. *Chemical Exposure* (Chapter 4)

   A. Pesticide
   B. Other

4. *Changes in Stress Levels* (Chapter 4)

  A. Recent Marriage
  B. Change in Residence
  C. Job Change (location or conditions, e.g., new boss, different duties)
  D. School Change
  E. Diagnosis of Serious Health Problem in Self, Family Member, or Close Friend
  F. Serious Loss (death, breakup, or other)
  G. Change in Household Composition (members join or leave residence)
  H. Relationship Problems
    Abusive Relationship
    Difficulty with Elderly Parent, In-Law, or Teenager
  I. Other

5. *Schedule Changes* (Chapter 4)

  A. Sleeping Times
  B. Meal Times

6. *Change in Exercise Regimen* (Chapter 4)

7. *Began/Stopped Computer Use* (Chapter 4)

8. *Weight Loss Programs* (Chapters 6 and 9)

  A. Packaged Meals/Supplements
  B. Use of Aspartame (NutraSweet™ or Equal™)
  C. Use of Appetite Suppressants (amphetamines)

9. *Other Dietary Changes* (Chapters 5 and 6)

   A. Low Fat Diet (emphasizing beans/oat products)
   B. Food Binges (e.g., chocolate)
   C. Vegetarian Diet (emphasizing beans, meat substitutes and/or cheese)
   D. Oriental Diet (frequent soy sauce, tofu, and/or MSG)
   E. Seasonal Changes
      e.g., Spring—Strawberries
      Holidays—Ham, Chocolate
      Other
   F. Change in Vitamin Intake

10. *Change in Caffeine Consumption* (Chapter 6)

   A. Coffee
   B. Tea
   C. Soft Drinks
   D. Medications

11. *Change in Nicotine Consumption* (Chapter 4)

   A. Source (cigarets, cigars, pipe, chewing tobacco, snuff, gum, or patch)
   B. Frequency

12. *Change in Alcohol or Cocaine Consumption* (Chapters 6 and 9)

   A. Type of Alcohol or Drug Used
   B. Frequency
   C. Amount
   D. Use of Antabuse (drug for treating alcohol abuse)

APPENDIX C

Natural Relaxation*

Preparation

Think of the next few minutes of "natural relaxation" as a pleasant time-out during the course of an otherwise busy day, rather than as another job to do. Since for the purpose of migraine control, you want to stay awake during this exercise, avoid using it right after a heavy meal or when you are extremely tired. Sit or lie down in a comfortable place (a recliner is ideal, but any soft chair or a bed with several pillows will do). Loosen any tight clothing, and leave your legs and arms uncrossed. Gently close your eyes.

Breathing

Be aware of your breathing now. Inhale slowly, feeling both your lungs and your abdomen expand; count to five before slowly exhaling. Again inhale, count, and exhale. Once more, breathe in, filling your lungs well. Now gradually release the air and the tension. Continue to breathe slowly and deeply. As you exhale, think to yourself: "This is *my* time."

*There are numerous variations of this progressive relaxation exercise, many involving deep breathing and the visualization of a pleasant scene. After you read through this version, you may want to record it for your personal use or to ask a friend with a pleasant voice to record it for you. Many migraineurs report success in preventing or aborting attacks by using similar exercises in the very early stages of an attack. And research suggests that the best results are obtained by people who practice their relaxation skills every day.

Once you feel comfortable with this version, you may want to consider getting a longer tape from a library or bookstore. Or you can lengthen this one or even produce an original. You should be successful just as long as you include these essential elements:

1. The deep breathing
2. Some form of the pleasant scene
3. The progressive relaxation
4. The return to present

About 20 minutes is considered the ideal time for achieving deep relaxation. Enjoy!

Pleasant Scene

Now imagine yourself in a very relaxing setting. It can be a place where you've actually been or where you've just wanted to go—either real or a total fantasy. Imagine what you are experiencing with your senses in this place: Does it feel warm or cool? Can you hear wind or water or other relaxing sounds? Are other people or possibly even animals there with you? In your mind's eye, picture yourself relaxing in this place; just enjoy it for a few moments.

Physical Relaxation

As you see yourself relaxing, you can feel the gentle movement of your own natural circulation in your feet. It is a very pleasant sensation.

This relaxing feeling spreads up from your feet to your legs; they are growing warm and heavy now. In your hips and abdomen you notice nerves and muscles begin to loosen. You are feeling pleasantly relaxed. Any tension that you might have felt during the day is slowly draining away.

Your back and shoulders are feeling comfortably relaxed now. It's almost as if your body is sinking into your chair.

Your scalp tingles pleasantly as if you've just brushed your hair. Any tightness in your neck is disappearing. You are becoming so relaxed that your head may even fall to one side. Your jaw, too, is very relaxed, and your mouth may even come open. That's okay; just enjoy the good feeling.

Your shoulders are very relaxed. They feel as if a kind friend with strong yet gentle hands has just massaged them. Your chest feels warm, heavy, and pleasant. This relaxing feeling spreads down your arms into your hands. Any remaining tension slowly flows down your arms and out of your body through your fingertips. Your arms and hands are very limber; in fact, they are as loose as an old spring that has lost all its tension . . . In your mind's eye, step back once again. View yourself as you are resting in your pleasant setting; just pause to enjoy it.

Returning to Present Awareness

To help you focus your attention back on the here and now, I am going to count to six; you will feel alert and refreshed after this brief relaxation exercise. One . . . two . . . begin to move your fingers and toes now; three . . . four . . . gently stretch your arms and legs . . . five . . . six . . . open your eyes now and return to your normal activities—relaxed but alert, with a sense of renewed energy.

APPENDIX D

Response Form
for Readers Exposed to Chlordane

Please photocopy this page
and mail to me at the address given below.

NAME:
ADDRESS:

Date(s) of chlordane exposure:

Situation (e.g., personal application; pesticide operator application; method and place of application, etc.):

Later change in migraine symptoms: Yes ___   No ___
    List specific change(s):

Interest in further networking: Yes ___   No ___

TO: Ms. Susan L. Burks
    PO Box 2083
    Newport News, VA 23609

APPENDIX E

Culinary Adaptations
From Susan's Kitchen

A Good Start

Breakfast Spiced Rice (1 serving)

Ingredients:

2/3 c. cooked brown rice (about 4 ounces)
1½ tsp. brown sugar
2 T. toasted wheat germ
1/2 tsp. cinnamon (or less, to taste)

a pinch of salt, nutmeg, or mace
1 egg white
1/4 c. milk
1 tsp. margarine, melted

Preparation: In microwave bowl, melt margarine. Add milk and egg white, and beat slightly. Add rice and dry ingredients and mix briefly to blend. Cover and microwave for 4-½ minutes on medium. (I cook large quantities of brown rice, keeping it refrigerated for several days or frozen indefinitely. Margarine can be added to rice while still warm from cooking, thus eliminating the need to melt and add later when making this cereal dish.)

Buckwheat Pancakes (2 servings or 6 medium-sized cakes)

Ingredients: 3/4 c. plus 1 T. Aunt Jemima Buckwheat Pancake Mix
3 T. toasted wheat germ
1/4 tsp. baking powder
1 whole egg plus one egg white, slightly beaten
2/3 c. skimmed milk
2 tsp. vegetable oil

Preparation: In medium-sized mixing bowl, briefly blend dry ingredients. Add beaten eggs with which milk and oil have been combined. Gently mix batter just until large lumps break up. Allow batter to "rest" for about 10 minutes while griddle heats. Cook on pancake griddle (heated to about 325 degrees) or in skillet. Serve with applesauce (preferably homemade) and cinnamon. Accompany with Gerber Meat Sticks that have been split lengthwise and broiled until light brown.

Simple Luncheon Fare

Greek Soup (1 serving)

Ingredients: 2 c. of homemade chicken stock*
1/4 tsp. garlic powder (or more or less, to taste)
3/4 oz. whole wheat noodles, uncooked
$2^1/_2$ oz. (about 2-1/2 c.) fresh spinach, washed and torn
    into bite-size pieces
3 oz. cooked chicken, cut into bite-size pieces
$1^1/_2$ tsp. white distilled vinegar
1/8 tsp. nutmeg
salt and pepper to taste

Preparation: In small saucepan with cover, bring broth and garlic to a
boil. Add noodles and simmer, covered, for 5 minutes; then add spinach and
continue simmering for 5 more minutes. Add chicken and heat briefly. Add
vinegar and sprinkle with nutmeg and salt/pepper, if desired. Ingredients
can be multiplied to make any amount desired.

Gourmet Baked Potato (1 serving)

Ingredients: 1 medium to large baking potato
1/2 to 2/3 c. low fat cottage cheese *without* added veg-
    etable gums; Breakstone, for example.
1/2 tsp. onion powder (plus a pinch for larger potato)
2 tsp. dried parsley (plus 1/2 tsp. for larger potato)
Salt, pepper, and margarine to taste

Preparation: Scrub and bake potato according to preference. (I like
using a conventional oven to get a crispy skin.) Split baked potato and add
margarine, salt, and pepper, if desired. Top with mixture of cottage cheese,
onion powder, and parsley.

Quick Rice Casserole (1 serving)

Ingredients: 2/3 c. cooked brown rice (with salt, pepper,
        and margarine to taste)
4 Gerber's Meat Sticks, each sliced into 4 pieces
1 T. gel from meat jar
1/2 tsp. onion powder
$1^1/_2$ tsp. dried parsley

Preparation: Briefly mix ingredients in small microwave-safe bowl.
Cover loosely and microwave on medium about 2 minutes.

*This is far better if you have poultry gel, the concentrated defatted juices from
baked poultry, to use for about 1/3 of the stock called for.

What's for Dinner?

Chicken–Green Bean Casserole (2 servings)

Ingredients: 1¹/₄ c. cooked brown rice
6 oz. chopped, cooked breast of chicken
1/2 lb. fresh green beans, steamed for about 10 minutes, or until crisp tender
1/2 c. canned water chestnuts, sliced (about 2/3 of a small can)
1 c. thin white sauce, made with 2/3 c. milk and 1/3 c. chicken stock or gel
1 tsp. onion powder
1/4 tsp. salt
1/3 c. toasted almonds, chopped or sliced
1/2 c. canned crispy-style Chinese noodles
paprika to taste

Preparation: Make white sauce and add onion powder and salt. In medium-size mixing bowl, briefly mix all except last three ingredients. Transfer to oven-proof casserole dish and top with almonds, noodles, and paprika. Bake at 325 degrees for 30 minutes or until bubbly and golden brown on top. (Or leave off toppings and heat rice mixture in microwave; add toppings and brown very briefly under broiler; watch carefully to prevent burning.)

A Good Finish

Pumpkin Custard (6 servings)

Ingredients:
1 egg and 1 egg white, slightly beaten
1-16 oz. can pumpkin
1/3 c. sugar, plus 1 T.
3/4 tsp. ground cinnamon
1/2 tsp. ginger

1/4 tsp. cloves
1 small can skimmed evaporated milk
1 c. low-fat milk
1 pinch salt

Preparation: Preheat oven to 350 degrees. Combine ingredients in order given. Pour into oven-proof glass pie dish. Bake about 50 minutes or until knife inserted near center comes out clean. Cool and serve with graham crackers (and a smidgen of whipped cream, if you dare.)

Apple-Bread Pudding (6 generous servings)

Ingredients: 8 slices heavy-style whole wheat bread (such as Pepperidge
　　　　　　　　Farm or Arnolds Stone Ground)
　　　　　　　1/3 c. sugar
　　　　　　　1 tsp. cinnamon
　　　　　　　3/4 tsp. vanilla
　　　　　　　3 egg whites, slightly beaten
　　　　　　　1$^{1}/_{3}$ c. low-fat or skimmed milk
　　　　　　　1 T. margarine, melted
　　　　　　　2 c. chopped cooking apples, unpeeled

Preparation: In large mixing bowl, briefly combine egg whites, milk,
vanilla, and sugar to which cinnamon and salt have been added. Add bread
that has been cut or torn into cubes and melted margarine. Set aside to let
flavors blend for about 20–30 minutes. (Apples can be washed and chopped
during this time.) After about 15 minutes, preheat oven to 350 degrees. Prepare large pan of hot water into which baking dish will be set. Add apple to
bread mixture and pour into greased 13 × 9 inch ovenproof glass baking
dish. Set dish into pan of hot water and bake for about 45 minutes or until
set. Serve cold for best flavor, preferably a day after baking. In two days, it
probably will taste even better.

APPENDIX F

Food Charts

LEVEL I—Worst Offenders

Foods to avoid	Comments/examples
Cheese	All *except* American, Farmer's, creamed, and cottage
Alcohol	Especially red wine
Caffeine	In excessive amounts (no more than two 5 oz.-cups of coffee per day)
Chocolate	All forms, including milk
Citrus	Grapefruit, lemons, limes, and oranges
Cured meats	Bacon, ham, all types of sausage, including pepperoni, hot dogs, and deli meats
Legumes	Broad beans, such as kidney, navy and others; lentils, peas, peanuts, and soy
Monosodium glutamate (MSG)	Especially bouillon, commercial soups and gravies, prepared entrees, and most canned tuna *See* notes on pages 88–90 for other common sources
Aspartame (Nutrasweet™/ Equal™)	In many artificially sweetened commercial products, such as soft drinks, desserts, and so forth

LEVEL II—Potent Headache Provokers

Food group	Item restricted
Beverages	Alcohol; chocolate milk and cocoa; coffee, sodas (brown and others containing caffeine), and tea; Ovaltine and Postum; ginseng
Cereals	All-bran, added bran (any grain), malt-flavored
Dairy products	Buttermilk, cheese (all except American and cottage), sour cream, and yogurt
Fruits and juices	Citrus, dried (all including coconut), grapes, Maraschino cherries, melon, papayas, pineapple, plums, raspberries, and strawberries
Protein	Cured meats (bacon, Canadian bacon, cold cuts and most deli meats, corned beef, ham, pressed turkey and turkey roasts, sausage, including pepperoni); dried, smoked, or pickled meat and fish (including barbeque, caviar, and anchovies); cold-water fish (such as tuna and salmon); marinated meats; organ meats (including all kinds of liver); and prebasted poultry. Peanuts and peanut butter; soy protein (including hydrolyzed vegetable protein or HVP)
Vegetables	Avocados and guacamole, broad beans (including pole, Italian broad, garbanzo, navy, white, lima,butter, and kidney), eggplant (especially the peel), garlic, lentils, mushrooms, onions, peas (black-eyed, green English, sugar snap, and snow), potato products containing sulfites (some canned, dried, and frozen), red cabbage, sauerkraut and tomatoes
Condiments	Commercial salad dressings, barbeque sauce, catsup, and mustard (except in very small quantities); pickles and olives; sauces (soy, terriyaki, worcestershire, or steak); vinegar (all except white distilled)
Miscellaneous	Aspartame (Nutrasweet™/Equal™); chocolate, carob (a chocolate substitute); commercial ice cream, pudding, and cottage cheese thickened with vegetable gums; natural licorice; malt; papaya-based meat tenderizers; seaweed/carrageenan; sourdough bread; soy flour; yeast extracts (like Marmite); any commercially prepared foods with unknown ingredients (hidden MSG)

LEVEL III—Generally Safe Foods

Food group	Types
Beverages	Water only
Cereals/grains	Rice only
Condiments	Salt, distilled white vinegar, vegetable oil
Fruits	Apples, peaches, and pears (peeled)
Protein	Very fresh beef, lamb, and chicken*
Vegetables	Beets, bell peppers, carrots, celery, cucumber, iceberg lettuce (discard outer leaves), potatoes (peeled), radishes, rutabagas, squash (all varieties), turnips

*If you are allergic to milk, eliminate beef; if allergic to eggs, avoid chicken.

APPENDIX G

Are You Ready
for Preventive Medication?

Write yes or no at the end of each statement.

1. *Adverse Effect on Personal Life:*

> I have at least two attacks per month. _____
> Attacks usually last longer than one day. _____
> Attacks often require bed rest. _____
> Attacks interfere with job performance or threaten advancement. _____
> I hesitate to make plans/commitments for fear of an attack. _____
> I am extremely upset about the frequency or severity of my attacks. _____

2. *Negative Impact on Significant Others:*

> Others complain about having to assume an unfair share of family/household responsibilities. _____
> I believe my attacks keep me from being the loving mate/parent/friend that I would like to be. _____
> If I were my significant other, I would resent these attacks. _____

3. *Appropriate Medical Attention:*

> I have had a thorough medical exam—including a manual examination of my neck and scalp areas—and have received a specific migraine diagnosis. _____
> I have informed my doctor about all other symptoms, conditions, and medications, and have asked about their possible effect on migraine. _____
> If female, I have charted my attacks to identify their possible relationship with my menstrual cycle and have shown this chart to my physician. _____

I do not abuse pain-relieving or migraine-abortive medications. _____

If I have allergy triggers, I have received appropriate medical
care for my allergies. _____

My attacks are either becoming less contained or are failing to
respond to abortive medications. _____

Medications that used to help my symptoms are becoming less
effective or are causing unpleasant side effects. _____

4. *Lifestyle Modifications:*

I have adopted regular eating and sleeping schedules, avoiding
missed meals and extreme fatigue. _____

I have not used tobacco products for at least six weeks. _____

I have given a migraine diet, including the elimination of
alcohol and caffeine, a serious trial for at least six
weeks. _____

I participate in regular aerobic exercise. _____

I have learned relaxation or biofeedback skills. _____

I have learned healthier coping mechanisms and have minimized
stress in all areas of my life. _____

I have minimized chemical exposures, including engine exhaust
and second-hand smoke. _____

I avoid or protect against glare/bright lights. _____

Overall Evaluation

A. Did you answer yes to two or more items in Sections 1 and 2 above?

B. Did you answer yes to all medical questions in Section 3 above?

C. Did you answer yes to all lifestyle questions in Section 4 above?

If your responses to A through C above are positive, then you may be
ready to consider taking preventive medication.

NOTE: Parts 3 and 4 of this questionnaire can be used to evaluate the
thoroughness of a migraine prevention program even if use of regular medication is not being considered.

APPENDIX H

Summary of Popular
Migraine Medications

The following material is intended for general information only. Please consult your personal doctor before beginning or changing medication, whether prescription or nonprescription.

Migraine Abortives

There is strong evidence that overuse of these drugs gradually leads to worsening of symptoms and in some cases even requires medically supervised withdrawal. Therefore, important dosage restrictions are included (courtesy of Dr. Sheftell).

Nonsteroidal Anti-Inflammatories (NSAIDs)*

Effectiveness: Highly effective; but considerable individual variation exists among patients, and experimentation may be required to find best drug choice. Particularly useful in menstrual migraine, when they can be taken regularly during the most vulnerable phase of the cycle, usually not more than one week per month.

Not Appropriate For: Patients with gastrointestinal symptoms, such as ulcers or bleeding, or those with significant kidney failure.

Use with Caution: In patients over 60, who as a group seem to be more susceptible to intestinal bleeding; those with high blood pressure, either untreated or treated; and those on other blood thinners.

Side Effects: Most common—gastrointestinal irritation/bleeding. (This may be "silent," i.e., without obvious symptoms.) Others vary according to drug; see package insert, or consult pharmacist or PDR.

Comments:

1. *May be used as both migraine preventives and abortives.
2. Take with food or milk.
3. Large initial doses may be needed when used as abortives.

4. With prolonged use, kidney function should be monitored and stool samples checked for blood.

5. Regular use may interfere with certain blood pressure medications, including beta blockers and the new drug Vasotec.

Restriction: No specific ones *provided all precautions are followed.*

Butalbital Combinations

Effectiveness: High, but abuse potential is also great and drowsiness can be disabling.

Not Appropriate For: Pregnant/nursing women; those who have trouble controlling alcohol and/or other sedatives; those who are allergic to any of the ingredients. (Codeine and aspirin are common allergens.) Aspirin should be avoided by persons who have ulcers or intestinal bleeding or who react with gastrointestinal distress.

Use With Caution: In persons with a family history of alcohol or drug abuse. In women using oral contraceptives (birth control effectiveness may be decreased).

Side Effects: Drowsiness, depression; eventual addiction if overused. Codeine is very constipating and may cause nausea and dizziness. Aspirin is a potent gastrointestinal irritant.

Individual Drugs:

Brand Name	Ingredients
Esgic, Fioricet,* and Repan	Butalbital, acetaminophen, caffeine
Fiorinal,* Fiorgen, Lisollyl, Lanorinal, and Marnal	Butalbital, aspirin, caffeine
Phrenilin	Butalbital and acetaminophen

Restriction: Two doses per attack, three times a week. If codeine is included, no more than 16 tablets a month. * Both of these products are also available with codeine.

Midrin/Isocom (Isometheptene Mucate, Acetaminophen, and Dichloralphenazone)

Effectiveness: Good for mild to moderate attacks.

Not Appropriate For: Pregnant/nursing women.

Use With Caution: In patients with severe circulatory problems or fever of any origin.

Side Effects: Generally well tolerated, but may cause dizziness.

Comments: Can be used alternatively with NSAIDs to prevent overuse of either drug.

Restriction: Two doses (two capsules each) per attack, no more than three times a week.

Ergot Derivatives

Effectiveness: High initially, but may decrease with use.

Not Appropriate For: Pregnant/nursing women, patients with heart disease, high blood pressure, or lupus, or those over 60 years.

Use With Caution: If fever is present, consult physician before using. *See* page 157 for special precautions to be taken with patients exhibiting certain risk factors.

Side Effects: Common—nausea and/or vomiting. Less frequent—rebound headache, cramping, restlessness, and hallucinations. Overuse can lead to chronic daily headache and serious circulatory problems. More serious side effects may include chest pressure or pain. If these occur, consult your doctor before using again.

Comments: Well tested; traditional drug of choice for severe attacks. If combined with caffeine (Wigraine/Cafergot), lower doses may be effective and side effects reduced.

Individual Drugs:

Brand Name	Administration	Dosage Range
Cafergot, Wigraine	Mouth	1 or 2 tablets; may repeat dose in one hour if needed
Cafergot	Suppository	1/4 to 1; may repeat in one hour if needed. Limit 2 doses per attack
Ergomar, Ergostat	Sublingual (dissolve under tongue)	1 Tablet; may repeat in 30 min. Limit 2 per attack

Restriction: Use no more than twice a week, two doses per attack, or follow your doctor's recommendation if the latter is more restrictive. Patients who need ergotamine more frequently may be "candidates for prophylactic therapy," according to Dr. Sheftell. However, he goes on to point out that this medication usually can be used safely and effectively for 3–5 days out of the month to combat menstrual attacks.

Imitrex (Sumatriptan)

Effectiveness: 81% rapidly helped by injection, somewhat fewer from oral dosing.

Not Appropriate For: Pregnant/nursing women; children under 16. Those with certain types of heart conditions, uncontrolled high blood pressure, or history of stroke. Patients who have used DHE or ergot products within the previous 24 hours.

Use With Caution: In those with decreased kidney or liver function or with a high risk of heart disease or stroke.

Side Effects: Generally minor; may include weakness, dizziness, and flushing, feelings of tingling, tightness, heaviness, pressure, and warmth. With the injectable form, localized burning, stinging, and brief pain have been reported. Rarely, nausea/vomiting. (During trials a few isolated cases of coronary artery spasm were reported.)

Comments:

1. Selectively constricts blood vessels in the head.
2. Relief is usually obtained within minutes to several hours, but headache may recur within 24 hours.
3. Available with autoinjector for simple at-home use.
4. A second 6 mg dose may be used after two hours if relief is partial.
5. Dr. Sheftell recommends that his patients try Imitrex during four attacks before judging it a failure.
6. Little is known about long-term side effects, including possible tendency to produce rebound headache.

Restriction: A maximum of two 6 mg injections within a 24-hour period; use no more than three times a week, a total of six injections per week.

DHE-45 (Dihydroergotamine Mesylate)

Effectiveness: Traditional drug of choice for interrupting the severe attack, usually in a medical setting. Clinical use generally has been positive.

Not Appropriate For: Pregnant women and patients with high blood pressure, heart disease, and liver or kidney malfunctions.

Side Effects: Nausea/vomiting (more common from IV dosage than from injection); less common—leg cramps/weakness, abnormalities in heart rhythm. Chemically different from ergot derivatives, this drug is less likely to cause rebound headache.

Comments:

1. An antinauseant usually is given first, but this may be unnecessary, especially if patient is not nauseated.
2. Can be taken by injection (patient can learn to do at home), or by IV in a hospital or emergency room.

Restriction: Weekly dose should not exceed 6 mg.

Corticosteroids

Effectiveness: High; used in severe, unresponsive attack or when ergotamine cannot be used.

Not Appropriate For: Pregnant/nursing women. Those with diabetes, glaucoma or lupus; those with heart, kidney, liver, or thyroid disease; those with high blood pressure, or active or inactive tuberculosis.

Side Effects: Fluid retention; flushing; may contribute to osteoporosis (especially prevalent in Caucasian/Oriental females with small bones).

Individual Drugs: dexamethasone, 4–6 mg given by mouth and followed in 3–4 hours by 2–4 additional mg if needed; *prednisone,* 20–40 mg, followed by 20 mg if needed.

Restriction: Use no more than once a month.

Antinauseants

Prescription Varieties

Generic	Brand Name	Comments
Chlorpromazine (by mouth, suppository, injection, or IV)	Thorazine	Usually well tolerated; may cause drowsiness
Metoclopramide (by mouth, injection or IV)	Reglan	Relative safety confirmed by wide use in British clinics
Prochlorperazine (by mouth, suppository, injection or IV)	Compazine	May cause dry mouth or sedation
Promethazine (by mouth or suppository)	Phenergan and others	Sore throat, bleeding, or unusual symptoms should be reported to physician

Effectiveness: Very high, either alone or in combination with other abortives. (*See* Chapter 10, pages 162–164, for more information about using these drugs alone rather than in combination as they usually are given.) In combination treatments, antinauseants are given 15–30 minutes before other medications in order to increase absorption.

Not Appropriate For: Pregnant/nursing women. Do not use alcohol, sedatives, tranquilizers, or barbiturates (butalbital combinations, for example) when taking the prescription varieties of these drugs.

Use With Caution: In those with glaucoma, epilepsy, ulcers, or difficulty passing urine.

Side Effects: Restlessness, involuntary muscle movements, possible seizures (rare).

Comments: Benedryl can be used to stop undesirable side effects.

Over-the-Counter—Emetrol
(Fructose, Dextrose, and Phosphoric Acid)

Effectiveness: Not established in controlled trials (Dr. Sheftell uses with some patients).

Not Appropriate For: Those with fructose intolerance (usually heredi-tary/runs in families).

Side Effects: Usually well tolerated.

Comments: Can be taken at home 20–30 minutes before other medica-tion, especially if nausea is prominent in attacks and is not controlled by the usual abortives/pain relievers.

Preventives

These drugs commonly are reserved for patients whose symptoms cannot be controlled successfully with abortive medication alone. (*See* Appendix G to focus on personal appropriateness of preventive medication.) Because these usually must be taken daily (or in the case of menstrual migraines up to one week per month), they tend to cause unpleasant side effects unless great care is paid in selecting both drug *and* dosage. In order to avoid over-dosing, patients should start on the lowest possible effective dose and then gradually increase as necessary. Dr. Sheftell provides the starting doses listed in the following section.

Beta Blockers

Effectiveness: A 25–50% improvement in the two-thirds who respond. Especially appropriate in those with angina and/or high blood pressure.

Not Appropriate For: Pregnant/nursing women, congestive heart patients, asthmatics, insulin-dependent diabetics.

Use With Caution: In those with depression, severe allergies, hypogly-cemia, insomnia, impotence, and Raynaud's Syndrome.

Side Effects:

1. General—interference with aerobic fitness and increase in undesirable blood fats (triglycerides and LDL, the bad cholesterol).
2. Central nervous system—depression, sleeplessness, memory loss, fatigue/weakness, loss of sexual desire.
3. Circulatory/respiratory—decreased blood flow in hands and feet, con-stricted respiratory passages, and impotence.

Comments:

1. Don't discontinue medication without directions from doctor.
2. May lose effectiveness after several years.
3. Some members of this drug family (those with sympathomimetic activity) that are useful in treating other conditions are *not* effective against migraine.

Individual Medications:

Generic	Brand Name	Comments
Propranolol*	Inderal	Most widely used/tested May cause all side effects listed
Timolol*	Blocadren	Similar to Inderal
Metoprolol**	Lopressor	Less likely to cause respiratory/circulatory side effects
Nadolol†	Corgard	Lowers triglycerides instead of raising them. Less likely to cause CNS side effects
Atenolol‡	Tenormin	Less likely to cause either respiratory/circulatory or CNS side effects

*FDA approved for migraine prevention.
**At doses below 200 mg/day, may be safer than some other beta blockers for patients with allergies, impotence, and Raynaud's Syndrome.
†At doses below 200 mg/day, may be safer than some other beta blockers for patients with depression, insomnia, and digestive disorders.
‡At doses below 200 mg/day, may be safer than most other beta blockers for many patients.

Starting Doses

Propranolol—20 mg twice a day (switching to the long-acting form only if 60 mg dose is needed)
Timolol—5 mg
Metoprolol—one-half of a 50-mg tablet
Nadolol—20 mg
Atenolol—one-half of a 25-mg tablet

Calcium Channel Blockers

Effectiveness: Controversial. May be very useful in patients with angina and/or high blood pressure and/or those who cannot take beta blockers, especially asthmatics and Raynaud's Syndrome sufferers.

Not Appropriate For: Pregnant/nursing women; those with very low blood pressure.

Side Effects: Constipation, fluid retention, fatigue, dizziness, nausea, and possible headache (either mild or severe).

Comments: Full benefits may not be realized for two months or longer.

Individual Medications:

Generic	Brand Name	Comments
Verapamil	Calan/Isoptin	Most widely used*
Diltiazem	Cardizem	Can interfere with heart rhythm (rare)**
Nifedipine	Procardia	A potent vasodilator; may cause daily headache[†]
Nimodipine	Nimotop	A potent vasodilator; may cause daily headache[†]

*Not appropriate for patients with liver damage.
**Not appropriate for patients with congestive heart problems.
[†]Using timed-release form may prevent/minimize this reaction.

Starting Doses: Verapamil—40 mg, 3 times a day, diltiazem—30 mg, 3 times a day, nifedipine—10 mg

Antidepressants

Tricyclics

Effectiveness: About equal to beta blockers, i.e., 25–50% improvement. Often combined with beta blockers if one drug alone is ineffective, or to keep dose of each low and thus minimize side effects.

Not Appropriate For: Pregnant/nursing women.

Use With Caution: In heart or stroke patients, those with liver damage, epilepsy, some types of glaucoma, thyroid disease, or difficulty in passing urine (enlarged prostate in men).

Side Effects: Common—dry mouth, constipation, weight gain, fatigue, and increased susceptibility to sunburn. Less common—changes in blood sugar, blood pressure, and sexual response.

Comments:

1. May not be fully effective for 2–8 weeks.
2. Smoking and vitamin C supplements may decrease effectiveness.
3. Alcohol should not be consumed while on these medications. (To his patients who insist on drinking, Dr. Sheftell advises no more than one

glass of wine with dinner and skipping the next dose of medication if any influence of alcohol remains; at least 6 hours should separate alcohol consumption and medication.)

4. Dental exams should be obtained at least twice a year to guard against gum disease.

Generic	Brand Name(s)	Comments
Amitriptyline	Elavil, Endep, etc.	Most widely used; drying effects most likely
Doxepin	Sinequan/Adapin	Sedating/drying
Imipramine	Tofranil, etc.	Less sedating/drying
Nortriptyline	Pamelor	Less sedating/drying
Desipramine	Norpramin	Least sedating/drying

Starting Doses: 10 mg at bedtime for each of the drugs listed above; Endep is scored in case a still lower starting dose is desired.

Monoamine Oxidase Inhibitor—Nardil (Phenelzine)

Effectiveness: High; useful in those who are severely depressed but who cannot take/fail to respond to tricyclics.

Side Effects: Dizziness (from low blood pressure), weight gain, possible hypertensive crisis.

Not Appropriate For: Patients who are unable or unwilling to follow complex instructions.

Comments:

1. Patients must avoid alcohol, certain foods, and medications.
2. Sometimes combined with tricyclics in severely depressed patients or to prevent hypertensive crises from certain foods and/or medications.

Starting Dose: 15 mg in the morning, gradually increasing to 45–90 mg, all to be taken before 3 PM.

Serotonin-Uptake Inhibitors—Prozac (Fluoxetine), Zoloft (Sertraline), and Paxil (Paroxetine)

Effectiveness: Not firmly established; early trials very promising. Helpful for those avoiding side effects of the tricyclics, especially weight gain and dry mouth.

Side Effects: Anxiety, sleep problems, bizarre dreams, daily headache, gastrointestinal irritation, diarrhea, low blood sugar: less common—loss of appetite/weight, decreased sexual desire/response. These may indicate an excessive dose.

Comments:

1. Should be taken with food or milk to avoid heartburn/other gastrointestinal irritation.
2. Alcohol should not be consumed while on this medication. (To his patients who insist on drinking, Dr. Sheftell advises no more than one glass of wine with dinner and skipping the next dose of medication if any influence of alcohol remains; at least 6 hours should separate alcohol consumption and medication.)
3. Gum disease may occur; dental exams should be obtained at least twice a year.

Starting Dose: 5 mg (liquid is available for ease of dosing or 10 mg capsule can be put into juice or food).

Sansert (Methysergide Maleate)*

Effectiveness: Some relief in 50–60% users. Some doctors reserve for severe sufferers who fail to respond to other preventives.

Not Appropriate For: Pregnant/nursing women.

Side Effects: Rare—long-term use causes dangerous circulatory problems and/or scar tissue formation in the chest or abdomen. More common—depression, fluid retention, muscle cramps, and abdominal discomfort.

Comments:

1. *FDA approved for migraine prevention.
2. To prevent complications, use for no more than 4 months continuously; then gradually decrease dose over about a week and wait 2–4 weeks before starting again. During this interval, X-rays or scans and blood tests should be used to check for any adverse effects.

Starting Dose: 2 mg daily for 3 days, increasing to 4 mg for additional 3 days, and finally 6–8 mg a day for remainder of recommended term.

Antihistamine—Periactin (Cyproheptadine Hydrochloride)

Effectiveness: High in children and those with menstrual migraine (used during the most vulnerable phase of the cycle).

Not Appropriate For: Pregnant women; those allergic to the phenothiazine family of drugs.

Use With Caution: In those with heart, liver, and stomach problems, or those wishing to avoid weight gain.

Side Effects: Sedation, increased appetite, weight gain, dizziness, dry mouth, sleeplessness, disturbed coordination; less common—itching, rash, sensitivity to sunlight, palpitations, headache, tremors.

Comments:

1. Use with alcohol and other sedatives and/or barbiturates likely to cause increased sleepiness and possible symptoms of depression.
2. Small doses at bedtime often both effective and well tolerated.

Starting Dose: 1/4 of a 4 mg tablet at night.

Analgesic—Stadol NS (Butorphanol Tartrate Nasal Spray)

Effectiveness: High for short attacks with severe head pain as primary symptom.

Not Appropriate For: Those under 18 years or with known opiate addiction problems.

Use With Caution: In those over 65; pregnant/nursing women; patients with respiratory, heart, liver, or kidney problems.

Side Effects: Short term—drowsiness, dizziness, nausea, and vomiting. Long term—nasal congestion, insomnia.

Dosage Restrictions: One spray in one nostril (1 mg); may be repeated in 60–90 minutes and again in 4 hours. Or, for the healthy patient between 18 and 65 years with severe pain, one spray in each nostril (2 mg); larger dose not to be repeated for at least 3 hours. Not to be used for more than two or three episodes a week in migraineurs.

Comments:

1. May cause addiction in long-term users.
2. Can interact with many other drugs, including alcohol and antihistamines.
3. Larger dose should not be used unless patient can lie down in anticipation of drowsiness/dizziness.

Suggested Readings/References

Chapter 1

Suggested Readings

Norman Cousins, *Anatomy of an Illness as Perceived by the Patient,* Norton, 1979.

Norman Cousins, *The Healing Heart: Antidotes to Panic and Hellessness,* Norton, 1983.

Norman Cousins, "The Patient-Physician Relationship," *Head First: The Biology of Hope*, Dutton, 1989.

H. Winter Griffith, MD, *Complete Guide to Medical Tests,* Fisher Books, 1988.

Antonio Van der Meer, "Diagnostic Dilemmas," in *Relief From Chronic Headache*, Dell, 1990.

Sidney Wolfe, MD and Rose-Ellen Hope, RPh, *Best Pills/Worst Pills: The Older Adult's Guide to Avoiding Drug-Induced Death or Illness,* Public Citizen's Research Group, 1993.

Betsy Wyckoff, *Overcoming Migraine,* Stationhill, 1991. (Contains list of headache clinics.)

References

E. Ian Adam, MD, "Migraine in General Practice," in *Migraine: Clinical and Research Aspects,* J. N. Blau, Ed., Johns Hopkins University Press, 1987.

J. N. Blau, MD, "Adult Migraine: The Patient Observed," in *Migraine: Clinical and Research Aspects.*

J. N. Blau, MD, "A Clinicotherapeutic Approach to Migraine," in *Migraine: Clinical and Research Aspects.*

Norman Cousins, *Head First: The Biology of Hope,* Dutton, 1989.

Seymour Diamond, MD, "Migraine Headaches,' in *the Medical Clinics of North America,* Seymour Diamond, Ed., Vol. 75, No. 3, 1991.

Steven Fraccaro, "Headaches," *American Health*, Vol. 10, 1991.

Edda Hanington, MD and Maurice Lessof, PhD, "Allergy," in *Migraine: Clinical and Research Aspects,* 1987.

Brian E. Mondell, MD, "Evaluation of the Patient Presenting with Headache," *The Medical Clinics of North America*, 1991.

Walter F. Stewart, PhD, et al., "Prevalance of Migraine Headache in the United States," *The Journal of the American Medical Association,* Vol. 267, No. 1, 1992.

Chapter 2

Suggested Readings

James W. Lance, MD, et al., "Contribution of Experimental Studies to Understanding the Pathophysiology of Migraine," in *Migraine: A Spectrum of Ideas*.

Joel R. Saper, MD, "Portrait of A Migraine," in *The World Book Health & Medical Annual*, World Book, 1989.

References

G. D'Andrea, MD, et al., "Platelet Norepinephrine and Serotonin Balance in Migraine," *Headache,* Vol. 29, 1989.

Seymour Diamond, MD, et al., "Migraine Headache—Working for the Best Outcome," *Postgraduate Medicine*, Vol. 81, 1987.

Vivette Glover, PhD and Merton Sandler, MD, "The Biochemical Basis of Migraine Predisposition," in *Migraine: A Spectrum of Ideas*, Merton Sandler, MD and Geralyn Collins, Eds., Oxford University Press, 1990.

Vivette Glover, PhD, et al., "Biochemical Predisposition to Dietary Migraine: The Role of Phenolsulphotransferase," *Headache*, Vol. 23, 1993.

John R. Graham, MD, "Discarded Therapies During the Past 50 Years" in *Migraine: Clinical and Research Aspects,* J. N. Blau, MD, Ed., Johns Hopkins University Press, 1987.

Edda Hanington, MD, "The Platelet Theory," in *Migraine: Clinical and Research Aspects*.

James W. Lance, MD, "Ten Thousand Years of Headache," in *Headache: Understanding, Alleviation,* Scribners, 1975.

Ninan T. Mathew, MD, "Transformed or Evolutive Migraine," in *Advances in Headache Research*, F. C. Rose, MD, Ed., John Libbey, 1986.

Kathleen R. Merikangas, PhD, "Genetic Epidemiology of Migraine," in *Migraine: A Spectrum of Ideas*.

Alan M. Rapoport, MD, "The Diagnosis of Migraine and Tension-Type Headache, Then and Now," in *Intractable Headache: Inpatient and Outpatient Treatment Strategies*, Supplement 2 to *Neurology,* Vol. 42, No. 3, 1992.

Alan M. Rapoport, MD and Stephen D. Silberstein, MD, "Emergency Treatment of Headache" in *Intractable Headache: Inpatient and Outpatient Treatment Strategies*.

Elliott A. Schulman, MD and Stephen D. Silberstein, MD, "Symptomatic and Prophylactic Treatment of Migraine and Tensiontype Headache," in *Intractable Headache: Inpatient and Outpatient Treatment Strategies*.

Fred D. Sheftell, MD, "Chronic Daily Headache," in *Intractable Headache: Inpatient and Outpatient Treatment Strategies*.

Seymour Solomon, MD and Richard Lipton, MD, "Criteria for the Diagnosis of Migraine in Clinical Practice," *Headache,* Vol. 31, 1991.

K. M. A. Welch, MD, "Migraine: A Biobehavioral Disorder," *Archives of Neurology,* Vol. 44, 1987.

Chapter 3

References

J. N. Blau, MD, "Adult Migraine: The Patient Observed," in *Migraine: Clinical and Research Aspects,* J. N. Blau, MD, Ed., Johns Hopkins University Press, 1987.

J. N. Blau, MD, "Loss of Migraine: When, Why and How," *Journal of the Royal College of Physicians of London,* Vol. 21, No. 2, 1987.

J. N. Blau, MD, "The Nature of Migraine: Do We Need to Invoke Slow Neurochemical Processes?, in *Migraine: A Spectrum of Ideas,* Merton Sandler, MD and Geralyn Collins, Eds., Oxford University Press, 1990.

John Edmeads, MD, "Four Steps in Managing Migraine," *Postgraduate Medicine,* Vol. 85, No. 6, 1989.

Edda Hanington, MD, "The Platelet Theory," in *Migraine: Clinical and Research Aspects.*

Edda Hanington, MD and Maurice H. Lessof, PhD, "Allergy," in *Migraine: Clinical and Research Aspects.*

R. C. Peatfield, MD, "A Note on the Role of Platelets in Migraine: A Personal View" in *Migraine: A Spectrum of Ideas.*

F. C. Rose, MD, "Trigger Factors and Natural History of Migraine," *Functional Neurology,* Vol. 1, No. 4, 1986.

George Selby, MD and James W. Lance, MD, "Observation of 500 Cases of Migraine and Allied Vascular Headache," *Journal of Neurological and Neurosurgical Psychiatry,* Vol. 23, 1960.

K. M. A. Welch, MD, "Migraine Pathogenesis Examined with Contemporary Techniques for Analysing Brain Function," in *Migraine: A Spectrum of Ideas.*

Chapter 4

Suggested Readings

John Bradshaw, *Homecoming: Reclaiming and Championing Your Inner Child,* Bantam Books, 1990. (Strategies for dealing with childhood stress that interferes with the adult present.)

Bette Hilleman, "Multiple Chemical Sensitivity," *Chemical and Engineering News,* July 22, 1991.

Jean Holroyd, PhD, "Two Exercises in Hypnosis," produced by *Psychology Today,* PO Box 78368, St. Louis, MO, 63178-9850 (1-800-444-7792).

Alan M. Rapoport, MD and Fred D. Sheftell, MD, "Letting Go of the Pain: Therapies and Relaxation Techniques," in *Headache Relief,* Simon and Schuster, 1990.

Steven M. Sack, *The Employee Rights Handbook,* Facts on File, 1991.

Joel R. Saper, MD, "Portrait of a Migraine," in *The World Book Health and Medical Annual,* World Book, 1989.

Jack Thrasher, PhD and Alan Broughton, MD, *The Poisoning of Our Homes and Workplaces,* Seadora, 1989. (Explores hazards of formaldehyde exposure and some possible avoidance strategies.)

Sidney M. Wolfe, Ed., "Carpet Chemicals May Cause Serious Health Risks," *Health Letter,* Public Citizen Health Research Group, March, 1993.

Grace Ziem, MD, "Diagnosing and Treating Chemically Injured People," *Pesticides and You* (The National Coalition Against the Misuse of Pesticides), Vol. 13, No. 2, Fall, 1993.

James Zinger, *Introduction to Self-Hypnosis,* Hypmovation Productions, 101 W. Alameda Ave., Burbank, CA 91502 (1-800-782-2333).

References

Alisa B. Arnoff, Esq., "New Law May Provide Job Protection," *National Headache Foundation Newsletter*, Summer, 1992.

J. N. Blau, MD, "Loss of Migraine: When, Why and How," *Journal of the Royal College of Physicians of London,* Vol. 21, 1987.

Mary Darling, "The Use of Exercise as a Method of Aborting Migraine," *Headache,* Vol. 31, 1991.

Seymour Diamond, MD, "Can Exercise Help Vascular Headache Sufferers?" *National Headache Foundation Newsletter*, Spring, 1992.

Rosemary Dudley and Wade Rowland, "Some Tips for Self-Help," and "The Triggers and How to Track Yours Down," in *How to Find Relief from Migraine*, Beaufort Books, 1982.

E. C. G. Grant, MD, Letter to the Editor, *British Medical Journal*, Vol. 287, 1983.

Edda Hanington, MD, "The Platelet and Migraine," *Headache,* Vol. 26, 1986.

Julia T. Littlewood, MSc, et al., "Migraine and Cluster Headache: Links Between Platelet Monoamine Oxidase Activity, Smoking, and Personality" *Headache,* Vol. 24, 1984.

Donna-Marie Lockett, MA and J. F. Campbell, PhD, "The Effects of Aerobic Exercise on Migraine," *Headache,* Vol. 32, 1992.

Susan McGrath (LA Times/Washington Post), "Household Environmentalist: Keep Formaldehyde Under Control," *The Birmingham News*, October 27, 1991.

Susan Menconi, MS, et al., "A Preliminary Study of Potential Human Health Effects in Private Residences Following Chlordane Applications for Termite Control," *Archives of Environmental Health*, Vol. 43, No. 5, 1988.

T. J. Payne, PhD, "The Impact of Cigarette Smoking on Headache Activity in Headache Patients," *Headache,* Vol. 31, 1991.

Joel R. Saper, MD, "Additional Conditions That Cause Headaches," in *Help for Headaches*, Warner Books, 1987.

Marjorie Shribman, Esq., "Obtaining Social Security Disability Benefits for Chronic Headache Sufferers," *National Headache Foundation Newsletter*, Summer, 1992.

Air Pollution in Your Home, American Lung Association Pamphlet, 1987.

Headache: Hope Through Research, National Institutes of Health Publication No. 84-158, September, 1984.

HOTLINE, "Chemical Sensitivity," *Motorhome*, August, 1991.

Chapter 5

Suggested Readings

Seymour Solomon, MD and Steven Fraccaro, *The Headache Book,* Consumer Reports Books, 1991.

References

B. Blackwell, E. M. J. Price, and D. Taylor, "Hypertensive Interactions Between Monoamine Oxidase Inhibitors and Foodstuffs," *British Journal of Psychiatry,* Vol. 113, 1967.

Katharina Dalton, MD, "Food Intake Prior to a Migraine Attack—Study of 2,313 Spontaneous Attacks" *Headache,* Vol. 15, 1975.

Seymour Diamond, MD, "Migraine Headache: Working for the Best Outcome," *Postgraduate Medicine,* Vol. 81, 1987.

Seymour Diamond, MD, Jordan Prager, MD, and Frederick Freitag, DO, "Diet and Headache: Is There a Link?" *Postgraduate Medicine,* Vol. 79, No. 4, 1986.

C. Gibb, MD, Vivette Glover, PhD, and Merton Sandler, MD, "Inhibition of PST-P by Certain Food Constituents," *Lancet,* i, 1986.

Vivette Glover, et al., "Biochemical Predisposition to Dietary Migraine," *Headache,* Vol. 23, 1983.

Patricia Guarnieri, Cynthia I. Radnitz, and Edward B. Blanchard, "Assessment of Dietary Risk Factors in Chronic Headache," *Biofeedback and Self-Regulation,* Vol. 15, No. 1, 1990.

Edda Hanington, MD and Maurice H. Lessof, PhD, "Allergy," in *Migraine: Clinical and Research Aspects,* J. N. Blau, MD, Ed., Johns Hopkins University Press, 1987.

R. J. Kohlenberg, PhD, "Tyramine Sensitivity in Dietary Migraine," *Headache,* Vol. 22, 1982.

M. H. Lessof, PhD and D. A. Moneret-Vautrin, "False Food Allergies: Non-specific Reactions to Foodstuffs," in *Clinical Reactions to Foods,* M. H. Lessof, Ed., Wiley & Sons, 1983.

Judy E. Perkin, RD, and Jack Hartje, PhD, "Diet and Migraine: A Review of the Literature," *Journal of the American Dietetic Association,* Vol. 83, 1983.

Chapter 6

Suggested Readings

George Schwartz, MD, "In Bad Taste: The MSG Syndrome," *Health,* 1988.

References

Steven Fraccaro, "Headaches," *American Health,* Vol. 10, 1991.

Claude A. Frazier, MD, "Allergenic Foods," in *Coping with Food Allergy,* Quadrangle, 1974.

Virgillio Gallai, MD, et al., "Serum and Salivary Magnesium Levels in Migraine," *Headache,* Vol. 32, 1992.

William Kropf, MD and Milton Houben, "The Twenty Worst Additives in Foods" in *Harmful Food Additives: The Eat Safe Guide,* Ashley Books, 1980.

Chris Lecos, "Reacting to Sulfites," *FDA Consumer,* Dec. 1985–Jan. 1986.

Lyndon E. Mansfield, MD, "Food Allergy and Headache," *Postgraduate Medicine,* Vol. 83, 1988.

Alfred L. Scopp, PhD, "MSG and HVP Induced Headache: Review and Case Studies," *Headache,* Vol. 31, 1991.

Chapter 7

References

Mary K. Beard, MD and Lindsay R. Curtis, MD, "Libido, Menopause, and Estrogen Replacement Therapy," *Postgraduate Medicine,* Vol. 86, No. 1, 1989.

K. Ghose, PhD, "Migraine, Antimigraine Drugs and Tyramine or Test," in *The Pharmacological Basis of Migraine Therapy,* W. K. Amery, MD, Ed., 1984.

Joe Graedon and Teresa Graedon, "The Next Miracles of Medicine," *The New People's Pharmacy,* Bantam Books, 1985.

John R. Graham, MD, "Discarded Therapies During the Past 50 Years" in *Migraine: Clinical and Research Aspects,* Johns Hopkins University Press, 1987.

Helen E. Hughes and Daniel A. Goldstein, "Birth Defects Following Maternal Exposure to Ergotamine, Beta Blockers, and Caffeine," *Journal of Medical Genetics,* Vol. 25, 1988.

James W. Lance, MD, et al., "Contribution of Experimental Studies to Understanding the Pathophysiology of Migraine," in *Migraine: A Spectrum of Ideas,* Merton Sandler, MD and Geralyn Collins, Eds., Oxford University Press, 1990.

E. A. MacGregor, MD, et al., "Migraine and Menstruation: A Pilot Study," *Cephalalgia,* Vol. 10, 1990.

G. Nattero, MD, et al., "Endocrine Aspects of Menopausal Migraine," in *New Advances in Headache Research,* F. C. Rose, Ed., John Libbey, 1988.

Richard P. Newman, MD, Letters to the Editor, "Clomiphene and Migraine," *Headache,* June, 1992.

Stephen D. Silberstein, MD and George R. Merriam, MD, "Estrogens, Progestins, and Headache," *Neurology,* Vol. 41, 1991.

Theodore L. Sourkes, PhD, "Influence of Hormones, Vitamins and Metals on MAO" in *MAO: Structure, Function and Altered Functions,* Thomas P. Singer, Ed., 1979.

Walter F. Stewart, PhD, et al., "Prevalence of Migraine Headache in the United States," *Journal of the American Medical Association,* January 1, 1992.

K. M. A. Welch, MD, "The Role of Estrogen in Migraine," *Cephalalgia,* Vol. 4, 1984.

Dewey K. Ziegler, MD and Arnold P. Friedman, MD, "Migraine" in *Merritt's Textbook of Neurology,* Lewis P. Rowland, MD, Ed., Lea & Ferbiger, 8th Ed., 1989.

Chapter 8

References

W. K. Amery, MD, "Cerebral Hypoxia and Migraine," in *Pharmacolological Basis for Migraine Therapy,* W. K. Amery, Ed., Pitman, 1984.

Michael Anthony, MD, "Unilateral Migraine or Occipital Neuralgia," in *New Advances in Headache Research,* F. C. Rose, MD, Ed., Smith-Gordon, 1989.

Charles Aring, MD, "Late-Life Migraine," *Archives of Neurology,* Vol. 48, No. 11, 1991.

Gunnar Bovim, MD, et al., "Neurolysis of the Greater Occipital Nerve in Cervicogenic Headache: A Follow-Up Study," *Headache,* Vol. 32, 1992.

Julie E. Buring, ScD, et al., "Low Dose Aspirin for Migraine Prophylaxis," *The Journal of the American Medical Association,* Vol. 264, No. 14, 1990.

Paul C. Davidson, MD and Harry K. Delcher, MD, "Hypoglycemia," in *Medicine for the Practicing Physician,* J. Willis Hurst, MD, Ed., Butterworth, 1983.

Seymour Diamond, MD, "Migraine and Depression," in *New Advances in Headache Research.*

John Edmeads, MD, "Migraine Equivalents and Complicated Migraine," in *The Medical Clinics of North America,* Seymour Diamond, MD, Ed., Vol. 75, No. 3, 1991.

John Edmeads, MD, "The Worst Headache Ever," *Postgraduate Medicine,* Vol. 86, No. 1, 1989.

C. M. Fisher, MD, "Late-Life Migraine Accompaniments as a Cause of Unexplained Transient Ischemic Attacks," *Canadian Journal of Neurological Sciences,* Vol. 7, 1980.

Vivette Glover, PhD and Merton Sandler, MD, "The Biochemical Basis of the Migraine Predisposition," in *Migraine: A Spectrum of Ideas,* Merton Sandler, MD and Geralyn Collins, Eds., Oxford University Press, 1990.

H. Winter Griffith, MD, "Cerebral Angiography," *Complete Guide to Medical Tests,* Fisher Books, 1988.

C. H. Gunderson, MD, "Management of the Migraine Patient," *American Family Physician,* Vol. 33, No. 1, 1986.

J. Littlewood, MD, et al., "Psychiatric Morbidity, Platelet Monoamine Oxidase and Tribulin Output in Headache," *Psychiatry Research,* Vol. 30, No. 1, 1989.

K. R. Merikangas, PhD and Jules Angst, MD, "Depression and Migraine," in *Migraine: A Spectrum of Ideas.*

K. R. Merikangas, PhD, et al., "Zurich Cohort Study of Young Adults," *Archives of General Psychiatry,* Vol. 47, No. 9, 1990.

J. E. Olsson, "Neuotologic Findings in Basilar Migraine," *Laryngoscope,* Vol. 101, Part 2, Suppl. 52, 1991.

W. J. Oosterveld, MD and L. I. Caers, PhD, "Antimigraine Drugs and Vestibular Function," in *The Pharmacological Basis of Migraine Therapy.*

F. C. Rose, MD, "Migraine Equivalents," in *The Prelude to the Migraine Attack,* W. K. Amery, MD, Ed., Saunders, 1986.

"Central Nervous System Infections," and "Nervous System Degenerative Dis-
    eases" in *The Clinical Practice of Neurological and Neurosurgical Nursing,*
    Joanne V. Hickey, RN, Ed., J. P. Lippincott, 2d Edition, 1986.
"Disorders of the Retina," in *The American Medical Association Encyclopedia of
    Medicine,* Charles B. Clayman, MD, Ed., Random House, 1989.
"The Eyes," in *Mayo Clinic Family Health Book,* David E. Larson, MD, Ed., Wil-
    liam Morrow, 1990.
"Radiopaque Agents," in *Advice for the Patient—Drug Information in Lay Lan-
    guage,* The United States Pharmacopeial Convention, 12th Ed., 1992.

Chapter 9

Suggested Readings

Norman Cousins, *Head First: The Biology of Hope*, Dutton, 1989.
Glen D. Solomon, MD, "Concomitant Medical Disease and Headache," in *Medi-
    cal Clinics of North America,* Seymour Diamond, MD, Ed., Vol. 75, No.
    3, 1991.

References

M. J. Biggs, BsC and E. S. Johnson, PhD, "The Automomic Nervous System and
    Migraine Pathogenesis," in *The Pharmacological Basis of Migraine Therapy*,
    W. K. Amery, MD, Ed., Pitman, 1984.
Vasant Dhopesh, MD, et al., "The Relationship of Cocaine to Headache in
    Polysubstance Abusers," *Headache,* Vol. 31, 1991.
A. Dhuna, MD, et al., "Cocaine Related Vascular Headaches," *Journal of Neuro-
    logical and Neurosurgical Psychiatry*, Vol. 54, No. 9, 1991.
P. Dostert, MD, "Requirements for New MAOI's," in *Monoamine Oxidase and
    Disease,* K. F. Tipton, Ed., Academic, 1984.
J. R. Fozard, MD, "5-HT in Migraine: Evidence from 5-HT Receptor Antagonists
    for a Neuronal Aetiology," in *Migraine: A Spectrum of Ideas*, Merton Sandler,
    MD and Geralyn Collins, Eds., 1990.
K. Ghose, PhD, "Migraine, Antimigraine Drugs and Tyramine or Test," in *The
    Pharmacological Basis of Migraine Therapy*.
Joe Graedon and Teresa Graedon, "A Practical Guide to Drugs of the 1980's" and
    "Behind the Scenes with OTC's," *The New People's Pharmacy*, Bantam
    Books, 1985.
Brian B. Hoffman, MD and Robert J. Lefkowitz, MD, "Catecholamines and Sym-
    pathomimetic Drugs," in *The Pharmacological Basis of Therapeutics,* Alfred
    G. Gilman, MD et al., Eds., Pergamon, 8th edition, 1990.
C. Raymond Lake, MD, et al., "Adverse Drug Effects Attributed to Phenyl-
    propanolamine: A Review of 142 Case Reports," *American Journal of Medi-
    cine,* Vol. 89, No. 2, 1990.
Chris Lecos, "Reacting to Sulfites," *FDA Consumer,* Dec. 1985–Jan. 1986.

R. C. Peatfield, MD and F. C. Rose, MD, "Exacerbation of Migraine by Treatment with Lithium," *Headache,* Vol. 21, 1981.

Theodore W. Rall, PhD, "Drugs Used in the Treatment of Asthma," in *The Pharmacological Basis of Therapeutics.*

Alan Rapoport, MD and Fred D. Sheftell, MD, "Drugs: Effects, Effectiveness, and Side Effects," *Headache Relief,* Simon and Schuster, 1990.

C. L. Ravaris, MD, et al., "Use of MAOI Antidepressants," *American Family Physician,* Vol. 18, No. 1, 1978.

S. L. Satel, MD and F. H. Gawin, MD, "Migrainelike Headache and Cocaine Use," *Journal of the American Medical Association,* Vol. 261, No. 20, 1989.

"Drugs Used for Psychogenic Disorders," and "Monoamine Oxidase Inhibitors" in *The Drug, The Nurse, the Patient* (Falconer's 7th Ed.), Eleanor Sheridan, RN, et al., Eds., W. B. Saunders, 1985.

Chapter 10

Suggested Readings

Alan M. Rapoport, MD and Fred D. Sheftell, MD, "Biofeedback: Learning to Monitor Yourself," *Headache Relief,* Fireside, 1991.

Sidney Wolfe, MD and Rose-Ellen Hope, RPh, *Worst Pills/Best Pills II: The Older Adult's Guide to Avoiding Drug-Induced Death or Illness,* Public Citizen Health Research Group, 1993.

References

W. K. Amery, MD, "Cerebral Hypoxia and Migraine," in *The Pharmacological Basis for Migraine Therapy,* W. K. Amery, Ed., Pitman, 1984.

Robert Bell, MD, et al., "A Comparative Trial of Three Agents in the Treatment of Acute Migraine Headache," *Annals of Emergency Medicine,* 10 Oct., 1990.

A. J. Bellavance, MD and J. P. Meloche, MD, "A Comprehensive Study of Naproxen Sodium, Pizotyline and Placebo in Migraine Prophylaxis," *Headache,* Vol. 30, 1990.

J. N. Blau, MD, "Adult Migraine: The Patient Observed," in *Migraine: Clinical and Research Aspects,* J. N. Blau, Ed., Johns Hopkins University Press, 1987.

J. N. Blau, MD, "Clinical Characteristics of Premonitory Symptoms in Migraine," in *The Prelude to the Migraine Attack,* W. K. Amery, Ed., Saunders, 1986.

David D. Celentano, et al., "Medication Use and Disability Among Migraineurs: A National Probability Survey," *Headache,* Vol. 32, 1992.

C. Dahlof, MD, "Flunarizine Versus Long-Acting Propranolol in the Prophylactic Treatment of Migraine," in *New Advances in Headache Research,* F. C. Rose, MD, Ed., Smith-Gordon, 1989.

Vincent DeQuattro, MD, Mark Myers, MD, and Vito M. Campese, MD, "Anatomy and Biochemistry of the Sympathetic Nervous System," in *Endocrinology,* Leslie J. DeGroot, MD, Ed., Saunders, 2nd Edition, 1989.

Seymour Diamond, MD, "Migraine Headaches," in *The Medical Clinics of North America*, Seymour Diamond, Ed., Vol. 75, No. 3, 1991.

John Edmeads, MD, "Four Steps in Managing Migraine," *Postgraduate Medicine*, Vol. 85, No. 6, 1989.

Frederick Freitag, MD and Seymour Diamond, MD, "The Longterm Use of Monoamine Oxidase Inhibitors in the Management of Headache," in *New Advances in Headache Research*.

Edda Hanington, MD, "The Platelet Theory," in *Migraine: Clinical and Research Aspects*.

H. Havanka-Kanniainen, MD, "Treatment of Acute Migraine Attack: Ibuprofen and Placebo Compared," *Headache*, Vol. 29, 1989.

K. A. Holyroyd, MD, et al., "Propranolol in the Management of Recurrent Migraine: A Meta-Analytic Review," *Headache*, Vol. 31, 1991.

Jeffrey Jones, MD, et al., "Randomized Double-Blind Trial of Intravenous Procholorperazine for the Treatment of Acute Headache," *Journal of the American Medical Association*, Vol. 261, No. 8, 1989.

H. D. Langohr, MD, et al., "Clomipramine and Metoprolol in Migraine Prophylaxis: A Double-Blind Crossover Study," *Headache*, Vol. 25, 1985.

H. G. Markley, MD, "Verapamil and Migraine Prophylaxis: Mechanisms and Efficacy," *The American Journal of Medicine*, Vol. 90, No. 5A, 1991.

N. T. Mathew, MD, "Drug-Induced Headache," *Neurological Clinics*, Vol. 8, No. 4, 1990.

Richard Peatfield, MD, "Drugs and the Treatment of Migraine," *Trends in Pharmacological Sciences*, Vol. 9, 1988.

A. Pradalier, MD, et al., "Non-Steroidal Anti-Inflammatory Drugs in the Treatment of Long-Term Prevention of Migraine Attacks," *Headache*, Vol. 28, 1988.

Hanna A. Saadah, MD, "Abortive Headache Therapy in the Office with Intravenous Dihydroergotamine Plus Prochlorperazine," *Headache*, Vol. 32, 1992.

P. S. Sorensen, MD, et al., "Flunarizine Versus Metoprolol in Migraine Prophylaxis: A Double-Blind, Randomized Parallel Group Study of Efficacy and Tolerability," *Headache*, Vol. 31, 1991.

Oksana Suchowersky, MD, "Rebound Headaches Due to Sumatriptan," *Neurology*, Vol. 43, April, 1993.

D. S. Tek, MD, et al., "A Prospective, Double-Blind Study of Metoclopramine Hydrochloride for Migraine in the Emergency Department," *Annals of Emergency Medicine*, Vol. 19, 1990.

Peer Tfelt-Hansen, H. D. Iversen, and Jes Olesen, MD, Letter to the Editors (Sumatriptan), *Journal of the American Medical Association*, Nov. 20, 1991.

Paul Turner, MD, "Beta-Adrenoceptor Blocking Drugs in the Prophylaxis of Migraine—A Critical Review," in *Migraine: Clinical and Research Aspects*.

Sidney M. Wolfe, MD and Rose-Ellen Hope, RPh, "Mind Drugs: Tranquilizers, Sleeping Pills, Antipsychotics, and Antidepressants," in *Worst Pills/Best Pills II*, Public Citizen Health Research Group, 1993.

Chapter 11

Suggested Readings

Norman Cousins, *Anatomy of an Illness as Perceived by the Patient,* Norton, 1979.
Norman Cousins, *Head First: The Biology of Hope,* Dutton, 1989.
Norman Cousins, T*he Healing Heart: Antidotes to Pain and Helplessness,* Norton, 1983.
William Glasser, *Positive Addiction,* Harper & Row, 1976.

References

Norman Cousins, "The Infinite Wonder of the Human Brain," and "The Laughter Connection," in *Head First: The Biology of Hope*, Dutton, 1989.
Seymour Diamond, MD, "Migraine and Depression," in *New Advances in Headache Research*, F. C. Rose, MD, Ed., Smith Gordon, 1989.
Vivette Glover, PhD and Merton Sandler, MD, "The Biochemical Basis of Migraine Predisposition" in *Migraine: A Spectrum of Ideas*, Merton Sandler and Geralyn Collins, Eds., Oxford University Press, 1990.
J. Jarman, et al., "Reduced Tyramine Sulphoconjugation in Migraine in Relation to Depression," in *New Advances in Headache Research*.
K. R. Merikangas, PhD and Jules Angst, MD, "Depression and Migraine" in *Migraine: A Spectrum of Ideas*.
K. R. Merikangas, PhD, Jules Angst, MD, and Hansruedi Isler, MD, "Zurich Cohort Study of Young Adults," *Archives of General Psychiatry*, Vol. 47, No. 9, 1990.
Guiseppe Nappi, MD, et al., "A New 5HT2 Antagonist in the Treatment of Chronic Headache with Depression: A Double-Blind Study Versus Amitriptyline," *Headache*, Vol. 30, 1990.
L. Teri and P. M. Lewisohn, "Group Intervention for Unipolar Depression," *Behavioral Therapist*, Vol. 8, No. 6, 1985.

Index